THE ATHLETE
INSIDE

THE ATHLETE INSIDE

The Transforming Power of Hope, Tenacity, and Faith

SUE REYNOLDS

Fortress Press

Minneapolis

THE ATHLETE INSIDE
The Transforming Power of Hope, Tenacity, and Faith

Cover image: FinisherPix®
Cover design: James Kegley

Print ISBN: 978-1-5064-5880-9
eBook ISBN: 978-1-5064-5881-6

DEDICATION

For my husband and sons.
I love how God is working in each of us.

To my husband, Brian:
God answered my prayers when he brought you into my life. Thank
you for your love and support for the past forty-plus years. You've
enabled me to chase big dreams with the confidence that you'd
always have my back if something went wrong. You are our family's
role model for everything good. I love you to the moon and back.

To my son Michael Dean:
Thank you for having the courage to open a meaningful discussion
in our family about God's love. You are truly a disciple of God,
and your gentle spirit allows others to open their hearts to you. I've
greatly enjoyed observing your passion for helping troubled youth as
you and Megan launch your Christian wilderness therapy program.

To my son Andy:
Thank you for pushing me to be healthy and for encouraging
me to do my first 5K. I love watching the joy you take in
your family and how you lovingly interact with your kids.
You and Laura are amazing parents. You've made a place
for yourself in the world of work, and your generous gift of
talent and time to your church and community is inspiring.

CONTENTS

Acknowledgments | ix

Introduction | 1

Before Triathlon | 7

8 → 335 → 235 pounds

Chapter 1: Becoming Obese | 9

Chapter 2: First Steps and Setbacks | 19

Chapter 3: Reset | 33

Triathlon Season 1: Crossing the Start Line | 43

235 → 226 pounds

Chapter 4: First Triathlon | 45

Triathlon Season 2: Discovering Me | 59

226 → 176 pounds

Chapter 5: Becoming Coachable | 61

Chapter 6: Facing Fear, Finding Courage | 75

Chapter 7: Discovering the Athlete Inside | 89

Chapter 8: I Know This Is You, God | 101

CONTENTS

Triathlon Season 3: Developing Grit | 113

176 → 140 pounds

Chapter 9: No Stone Unturned | 115

Chapter 10: Who Am I? | 133

Chapter 11: Team USA | 145

Triathlon Season 4: World Championship | 157

140 → 135 pounds

Chapter 12: Building the Team | 159

Chapter 13: Catastrophe, Faith, and Cozumel | 169

Chapter 14: Worlds! | 181

Triathlon Season 5: Sixth in the World | 199

135 pounds

Chapter 15: Blues and Joys | 201

ACKNOWLEDGMENTS

Losing two hundred pounds, becoming a triathlete, and writing a book about my journey have been possible through the love, support, and kindness of many people. In addition to those to whom I dedicated this book, I am immensely grateful for the following people who have played a part in my journey. Thank you, all of you.

My daughters-in-law, Laura Reynolds and Megan Reynolds: I love having other girls in the family, especially ones as sweet as you. You have blessed me beyond words by loving my sons.

My grandchildren, Harper, Emma Kate, Caroline, and Mack: You bring laughter and joy into our lives. You make my heart sing.

My brother and Ironman, Tom Engle: Although you are my little brother, you have always seemed like a big brother. I appreciate your wisdom (which I'm sure you inherited from Dad), all you've taught me about triathlon, and how you always know the right words to calm my nerves before big races.

Coach Brant Bahler: You saw things in me that I didn't know existed, helped me develop the confidence I needed to go after my dreams, and supported me every step of the way. Through your actions, you taught me how trust is built. Most importantly, you showed me how deep one's faith can be, helped me see the doors that God put before me, and helped me have the courage to step through those doors. I am grateful for your triathlon guidance, your silly sense of humor, and our intergenerational friendship.

USA Triathlon: Thank you for all your support and encouragement as I transitioned from a triathlon newbie to a member of Team USA. I will never forget your kindness.

Adam Schaeuble and the coaches at Next Generation Personal Training/Meltdown Bootcamp: I am grateful for the nutrition and exercise instruction I received at Bootcamp, along with Bootcamp's supportive culture and accountability system. Bootcamp was exactly what I needed to start my fitness journey.

Matt Fitzgerald: Your many books on nutrition for endurance athletes fill my personal library. Thank you for helping me determine my ideal race weight and for your personal interest in my story which gave me courage to share it with others.

My sports performance dietitian, Brittney Bearden: Your guidance, kindness, and patience as I transitioned from a weight loss nutrition plan to a sports performance nutrition plan were greatly appreciated. Your plan worked. I have sustained my ideal race weight for several years.

My writing mentor, John Woodcock: Your guidance and positive support as I wrote the first draft of each chapter meant so much to me. Your kind encouragement caused me to fall in love with writing. I will cherish that gift forever.

My literary agent, Julie Gwinn: I will never forget the shock I felt when I asked before writing a word of this book, if you thought anyone would be interested in reading it, and you replied, "Yes . . . and I'd like to sign you right now." Thank you for believing in me and for all the help you have given me along the way.

The team at Fortress Press: I appreciate all your editing, proofreading, designing, typesetting, producing, and promotion for the book. Emily Brower and others, thank you for guiding me through the editing process and for helping me understand that I can't have thirty-six exclamation points in one chapter!

And most importantly, thanks to God: You welcomed me back with open arms when I had been away and have showered me with abundant blessings for which I am deeply grateful. I pray that you will help me have the ability to recognize your will and the tools I need to put your will into action. While I may win a race or receive a medal, all glory goes to you.

INTRODUCTION

Yesterday, my emotions were a mess. But today, I feel surprisingly calm. I stand shoulder to shoulder with 113 of the fastest women my age from around the world. Together, we wait for the start of the International Triathlon Union's Age Group Triathlon World Championship ("Worlds" for short) in Cozumel, Mexico. I'm here because a year ago, the governing body for triathlon in the United States invited me to be a member of Team USA, based on my second-place performance at the Draft-Legal Triathlon World Qualifier in Clermont, Florida.

Large letters plastered across the front and back of my red, white, and blue uniform spell out REYNOLDS USA. Each of the women around me wears a similar skintight outfit in the colors of her country's flag and bearing her country's three-letter code. The woman next to me wears a green uniform with MEX written across the front. The woman next to her wears red, with JAP identifying her country. Looking around, I also see AUS, BER, CAN, GBR, NZL, and many others.

Today's race is one of several triathlon events that will occur over the next few days. At the end of the week, a medals count will be announced at the closing ceremony, with each country hoping for bragging rights. I feel incredible pride and excitement as I wait to race on behalf of my country. But then I shake my head in wonder. How is this possible?

Four years earlier, I was obese at 335 pounds. I couldn't walk a block or even stand without gasping for air. Sitting in a restaurant booth was out of the question; my large body wouldn't fit into the seat. When driving in friends' cars, I'd hear, "Ding! Ding! Ding!" and have to explain that I couldn't get the seat belt around my waist. I had no clue that I even liked sports and certainly had no idea an athlete was hiding inside my immense body.

Now, at the race, I listen to the women around me speaking in different languages, and I wonder if they are nervous. In a few minutes, we will all jump from a long dock built specifically for Worlds into the Gulf of Mexico. Our race is a sprint triathlon consisting of a 750-meter swim (0.5 miles), 20-kilometer bike ride (12.4 miles), and 5-kilometer run (3.1 miles). Unlike the longer Ironman triathlon, where participants progress at a steady pace for up to seventeen hours, competitive sprint triathletes race as fast as they can from start to finish. The winner in my age group will complete the course in about an hour and twenty minutes.

The challenge for competitive sprint triathletes is pushing through intense pain to a point just below redline, or the maximum exertion that the body can sustain, for the entire race. Mental strength is required to keep going fast when the body is screaming for relief. At the same time, sprint triathletes must be careful to not push so hard that their body shuts down. If that happens, no matter how hard they push, they will go slower and slower. Toward the very end of the race, when their body is exhausted, sprint triathletes push beyond redline to finish strong, hoping their body has enough gas left in the tank to carry them over the finish line. While some people prefer the longer and slower Ironman triathlons, I love the sprint distance.

As I wait with the other women for the start of our race, I reflect upon the last few years and feel dumbfounded. Four years ago, I had given up hope that I could be anything but morbidly obese. And just three years earlier, I finished second to last in my first local triathlon. Yet now I race on behalf of the United States against the fastest triathletes in the world. Unbelievable!

I savor the moment. Just being at Worlds is a dream come true. I think about how far I've come: the hopes and dreams; the tenacity it took to keep going when fear, pride, and exhaustion threatened to get in the way; and the spiritual journey I didn't expect. My eyes mist as I think about all of the people who believed in me and helped me along the way: my husband and family, who supported me from day one; my young coach, who saw things in me that I never imagined possible; and the perfect strangers who popped into my life at just the right moment, saying just the right thing to give me the courage I needed to move forward. The kindness of so many people touches my heart in the most profound way, and as I wait for the start of the race, I feel overwhelming gratitude.

My mind shifts, and I start thinking about the fears I conquered to get to Worlds. As a beginning triathlete, I was terrified by everything—swimming in a lake with fish, riding my bike on the road with cars, wearing a wet suit, clipping into my bike pedals, running up steep hills, the real possibility of injury. I also feared that my slowness would inconvenience the race volunteers who would have to wait for me to cross the finish line, long behind the other participants. Thankfully, I found the courage to face and overcome those fears.

I look at the women standing around me. Almost all of them have been racing for years and are proven triathletes. Some own sports shops, while others coach college-level sports teams. Some are previous world champions and all-Americans. In contrast, I am a novice with just three years of experience. For months, I've been using self-talk to build my confidence: *You are not out of your league. You deserve to be at Worlds. You earned this position.*

My start time gets closer. I shake out my arms and legs. I take some deep breaths. In spite of my previous fears, my nerves are now exactly where I want them. I am a little nervous but not overly so. I feel a quiet confidence. I know I am prepared. Now I just need to do the job I came to do.

Finally, the announcer calls our wave to the start, first in Spanish and then in English. My heart rate increases just a bit, and I take some deep breaths to slow it down. While I usually hang back as everyone lines up for the start of the race, this time I go straight to the front and jog confidently down the long, narrow dock that juts out into the Gulf of Mexico. All of the other women follow behind me. Suddenly, it hits me that I am leading a line of the best triathletes in the world to our starting positions for the Age Group Triathlon World Championship. The moment seems surreal, but this is actually happening. This is Worlds! Simultaneously confident and overwhelmed with excitement, I remain determined and focused as I lead 113 of the world's best triathletes to the start of the race.

I reach the end of the dock and see painted lines every eighteen inches or so along the left edge. They mark the athletes' starting positions. I run straight to the spot where I want to start, directly across from the first buoy. Then I stand for a few seconds, gazing over the water, soaking in the moment. My coach's calm words wash over me: "Trust your training. You are prepared. Follow the plan. You are a competitor." His last statement quickly becomes my mantra for the day, and I repeat it to myself over and over: *You are a competitor. You are a competitor. You are a competitor.* I am filled with confidence. I am ready.

After pressing my goggles tightly against my eyes, I jump into the warm water of the Gulf of Mexico. I swim a three-minute warm-up, and then, as directed by the starter, I place one hand on the dock above me. I think about all the hands lined up on that dock—the hands of the fastest triathletes in the world. Again, I'm filled with wonder. And then suddenly, the starter yells "Set!" I tense my body, prepare to spring into motion, and wait for the sound of the air horn.

• • •

My journey began when I read online about a woman who lost over a hundred pounds without drugs or surgery. I never met her, but her story gave me hope. If she could lose a hundred pounds, I could, too. My wish is that my story might instill in others similar hope that they can succeed in their own transformation journey. For some, the transformation may be personal—to lose weight, become fit, pursue a new level of education, earn a promotion, strengthen their faith, or be kind. For others, the journey may be about transforming an institution or even the culture of our society. Whatever the transformation, this I know to be true: with hope, tenacity, and faith, anything is possible.

BEFORE TRIATHLON

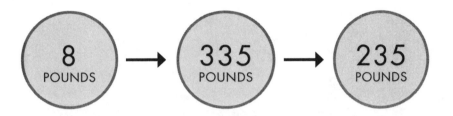

Chapter 1

BECOMING OBESE

I wasn't always obese. In fact, in preschool I was considered "thin enough" to model children's clothing at garden parties, where affluent women would examine the clothes I wore and tell me how cute I was. I learned at an early age that my appearance could be pleasing to people, and that made me happy.

During my time in middle school, ultrathin models like Twiggy started shaping the public's image of the perfect body. I continued to be thin and earned the title of runner-up for our school's homecoming queen.

My first memory of dieting comes from high school. I'd eat an orange for lunch and a can of Metrecal, a stew-like diet meal, for dinner. One of my brother's friends told him that he had a hot sister. I smiled as I saw my brother's pride. Once again, I found that my appearance could make people happy.

When I was in college, my mother told me that she dreamed I would have long, thin legs and arms along with an interest in art. In her dreams, I would marry a highly successful man, who would go off to work each morning while I stayed home doing art projects to fill my time. I didn't think marrying a rich man was important, but I did stay relatively thin and grew to love art projects. At the same time, I started to rebel. During the day, when my mother was out of the house, I'd make peanut butter and jelly sandwiches and hide them. At dinner, I'd eat the small portions that my mother served. But after dinner, I'd devour the peanut butter and jelly sandwiches I had hidden earlier in the day. Even with extra calories, however, my weight stayed relatively low.

After college, my weight started to increase as I began a career in education. I often stayed up all night grading papers and preparing for the next day's lessons. I loved teaching and happily worked long into the night. I quickly learned that eating helped me stay awake as I worked. The pounds started building on my five-foot, eight-inch frame, and I often skipped meals in an attempt to keep my figure slim.

I met my husband after I had been teaching for a couple of years. The school's chemistry teacher, Bob, had been pushing me to go out on a blind date with one of his friends. Bob predicted that the young man and I would fall in love and get married. I wasn't buying it. I had never been on a blind date and had no intention of meeting Bob's friend. Then one day, the phone rang, and Bob was on the other end. "Just a minute," he said.

A new voice came on the phone: "Um . . . hello. Um . . . this is Brian. Um . . . listen. Has Bob been bugging you to go out with me? Yes? Well, um, he's been bugging me about going out with you, too. So . . . um . . . let's just go out and get him off our backs." I agreed.

A few days later, Brian took me out to lunch. We talked about our lives and I learned that Brian had worked three jobs to put himself through college. Then we went for a drive in the country. When I told Brian that I had never driven a car with a stick shift, he immediately stopped the car and told me I was driving home. I slid behind the driver's wheel and sent the car into a series of lurches separated by halting stops. We rolled in laughter and I fell in love with Brian's silly side, his eagerness to take me on new adventures, and his patience. That was my first—and only—blind date. We married two years later. I walked down the aisle at 120 pounds, whispered into my Dad's ear, "I love you," and then stepped forward to begin life with Brian.

Brian was not the successful "catch" that my mother had envisioned me marrying. Before retirement, his father worked as a pipefitter, and his family didn't have the income that my family enjoyed. But the qualities that Brian possessed—integrity, kindness, loyalty, and determination—were much more valuable to me than the blue blood my mother sought. We've been married for over forty years, and he offers me unconditional love and respect every day.

As a new wife, I believed it was my job to fatten up my husband, who looked like a rail. I baked pies and cookies and really worked to put some meat on his skinny bones. The results were ironic: Brian gained three pounds, and I gained thirty. I now had two situations that challenged my waistline: eating to stay awake and cooking for my skinny husband. Slowly, my weight started to build.

The final blow in my battle with weight came from a new job. After working in public schools for ten years and then spending another ten years as a consultant for the Indiana Department of Education, I founded a nonprofit and began working as its president. My work didn't seem like a job. For me, it was a calling. We taught schools how to raise student achievement, especially for lower-income students, who didn't have the same supports and opportunities as their more privileged peers. I loved that we made a difference in the lives of young people. Work was a joy, and all-nighters became routine.

One (typical) night, I sat in my office on the first floor of our two-story home. My husband and our two sons slept soundly upstairs, and our dog snored quietly in the family room. It was 2:00 a.m., and all was well, except I had to finish writing a speech I would give the next morning. I faced another all-nighter, the third one that week. It sounds crazy, but I didn't mind. I was on a mission. I could catch up on sleep over the weekend.

From my years of teaching, I knew how to stay awake night after night. I went to the kitchen to find a snack that would keep me company during the long hours ahead. Preferably, I'd find something I could nibble on—chips, cereal, crackers, popcorn. I found a bag of chocolate chips. Bingo. Back at my desk, I worked for a while more, staying awake as my hands traveled between the computer, the chocolate chips, and my mouth. An hour later, I needed a break. I walked back to the kitchen to search for something that would keep me awake a while longer. I found ice cream in the freezer. Perfect.

As our nonprofit organization grew, so did my waistline. Over the years, I went from size medium to large to extra-large. Finally, I couldn't buy clothing in stores anymore and started ordering my wardrobe from online shops that sold big sizes. I went from XL to XXL and then to 3X, 4X, and 5X. I found it amusing that clothing manufacturers used abbreviations so they wouldn't have to write extra-extra-extra-extra-extra-large on their clothing tags. I also found fashion unavailable in larger sizes. My clothing now consisted of slacks with elastic waistbands and tunic tops that hung down to my thighs.

When I hit size 3X, I stopped looking at myself in the mirror other than to brush my hair in the morning. I forbade people to take pictures of me, and I stopped weighing myself. I didn't want to see evidence of the weight I had gained. Without mirrors or photos, I could see only my forearms and hands as they worked on the keyboard or put food in my mouth. Unlike the rest of me, they were slim. I had no real sense of how big I had become. I didn't want to know. Even when my doctor wrote on a report that I was morbidly obese, it didn't sink in. I told myself that since I had normal blood pressure, my obesity was not a health risk, and I put that out of my mind, too.

I also found that foods high in carbohydrates, like bread, potatoes, and sweets, helped to relieve stress. Those foods made me feel calm under pressure. When facing a deadline, I sought carbohydrates the way an addict turns to alcohol or drugs. As this became a habit, my size started to increase more and more. However, I had no idea how much weight I had gained. The more weight I gained, the more I didn't want to know how much I weighed.

Of course, my family became concerned for my health and well-being. My husband and sons repeatedly told me that I needed to lose weight. Often, my husband would gently remind me that I didn't need that sixth slice of pizza or third piece of cake. Before our first grandchild was born, our younger son suggested that if I lost weight, I'd be able to get down on the floor and play with my grandkids. When that didn't get through, he said very bluntly and firmly, "Mom. You are going to die. I want my children to have a grandma." It broke my heart that my son worried about me dying, but I shrugged off his concerns. Yes, I was a big woman, but my blood pressure was in the normal range. I was not going to die. I would be there for my grandchildren. I didn't need to lose weight.

I was wrong. The National Center for Health Statistics states that almost 40 percent of adults in the United States are obese, with obesity defined as a number of 30 or greater when dividing weight in kilograms by height in meters squared.[1] They also state that those suffering from obesity are more likely to develop diabetes, hypertension, stroke, arthritis, and certain types of cancer—some of the leading causes of preventable death.[2] My son was right. My obesity increased my chances of a potentially fatal condition and lessened the chance that my grandchildren would have a grandma. But at the time, I wasn't ready to accept that truth.

• • •

People sometimes ask how I developed into a person who is comfortable with big dreams and has the tenacity and grit to reach them often. I always point to the support of my parents and teachers. Their faith in me played a large role in helping me learn how to dream big and then work hard to reach those dreams.

My father's faith in me was especially key. I always adored my dad but didn't see much of him when I was growing up. As an executive engineer for Chrysler Corporation, he worked all day. After dinner, he went to his study to do paperwork that he brought home from the office. In my mind, my dad ran the automotive industry while my mother ran the family. But once in a while, my dad lifted me high in the air and put me on top of his shoulder "like a bag of potatoes" and carried me around as I shrieked with joy. Sometimes he'd sit on the side of my bed after tucking me in at night and ask, "Have any problems?" If I had a problem with a friend or at school, he always gave me wise advice and told me he had faith in me to handle the situation. While my dad's work kept him busy, he always took time to celebrate my accomplishments. We'd go out for dinner when I had a good report card, and once, when I won a little medal, he went to his workbench and made a plaque for displaying it.

My relationship with my mother was different, but her faith in me to succeed at a high level was clear. Like most moms at the time, she did not work outside of the home. Her job was to manage our family and teach my brother and me how to become productive, responsible adults. Before I was born, my mother worked as a chemist at Pratt and Whitney, which was pretty remarkable in the 1940s, when males dominated the field of chemistry. She was a pioneer and an achiever.

My mother always insisted that I perform at a high level and supported me so I could. Her drive and ambition taught me the value of grit and tenacity, even when I didn't want to learn. She made sure I did my homework from school and checked it each evening. We'd stay up late at night while she quizzed me before tests and wouldn't let me stop until I had mastered all the material. She told me she had eaten Cheerios in college to stay awake late into the night studying. She often brought me a bowl of ice cream when I was studying.

Sometimes, my mother's insistence on performance felt overwhelming. As a teenager, I once screamed at her, "Just let me fail!" But other times, her belief in me filled me with confidence and made me proud. When I started working as a first-year teacher, my mother told me I should become superintendent of public instruction for the entire state. I had no aspirations for climbing that career ladder, but it felt wonderful to know she believed in me. My mother's actions taught me to have big dreams, and her insistence on hard work taught me the discipline and consistency it takes to reach them. The little successes I experienced early in life taught me to love the deep satisfaction that comes with accomplishing a hard task.

My mother's actions also taught me to love the outdoors. When my brother and I were kids, she often sent us outside to play. I ran for the joy of running, climbed trees, built forts in the woods across the street, and explored faraway places on my bike. When I'm training for triathlon, I often feel as if I'm ten years old again, out in the neighborhood, playing with my friends.

While most of my lessons about dreams, hope, and tenacity came from my parents, others came from my teachers. My fourth-grade teacher, Mrs. Springer, helped me understand that I had the power to take on tasks much bigger than I thought possible. Once, when we were reading a novel that mentioned the Great American Desert, I became confused. A few days earlier, Mrs. Springer had taught us that deserts don't exist in the United States. Curious, I raised my hand and asked Mrs. Springer to clarify. Instead of answering, she suggested that I send my question to the book's publisher.

As a nine-year-old, I couldn't imagine writing to a publisher, but she encouraged me to do so and helped me compose the letter. Two weeks later, I was shocked when the publisher wrote back. All of a sudden, I wasn't a just an invisible little kid anymore. I was someone whose questions mattered. Mrs. Springer taught the joy of being curious and that it's OK to ask questions. Those lessons have served me well over the years. In triathlon, I bombard my coach with one question after another on a daily basis, so I can learn everything I can about swimming, biking, and running.

While my parents and teachers taught me to have big dreams and to work hard, I had to figure out which dream-reaching tools worked for me. When I needed to stay up late to complete a task or when things got stressful, food did the trick. With the help of cookies, chocolate, ice cream, and other sweets, I did the work that needed to be done to start and sustain a successful nonprofit that helps kids succeed in school. Food got the job done . . . for a while.

Notes

1. Craig M. Hales, Margaret D. Carroll, Cheryl D. Fryar, and Cynthia L. Ogden, "Prevalence of Obesity among Adults and Youth: United States, 2015–2016," NCHS Data Brief (National Center for Health Statistics), no. 288, October 2017, https://tinyurl.com/yxecx54z.

2. "National Health and Nutrition Examination Survey," NCHS Fact Sheet (National Center for Health Statistics), December 2017, https://tinyurl.com/y48azolx; CDC National Health Report Highlights, Centers for Disease Control and Prevention, U.S. Department of Health and Human Services, 2014, https://tinyurl.com/y4eh8g9h.

Chapter 2

FIRST STEPS AND SETBACKS

When I started losing weight, I wasn't planning to lose 200 pounds. I was just beginning another diet, as I had so many times over the years. At 335 pounds with endless failed diets behind me, I had high hopes but no real expectation that this time would be different. I assumed that history would repeat itself: I'd lose weight but then gain it all back, along with an additional 10 to 20 pounds. If I were to graph my weight over the years up to this point, it would look like a roller coaster with each peak a little higher than the one before.

But this time, something was different. My rationale for losing weight—my why—had changed. Having a strong why is important in any challenging journey. When the going gets tough, your why keeps you on track. In past diets, my why had been to please other people. As a child, I wanted please my mother, who told me I should be thin.

In middle and high school, I wanted to meet society's expectations conveyed by the skinny models I saw on TV. As an adult, I wanted to please my husband and sons, who urged me to be a healthy weight. However, pleasing people wasn't a strong enough why to keep me on course when I was working all night with chocolate chip cookies in the kitchen. In those situations, I'd put all the people who urged me to be thin out of my mind and eat one cookie after another.

Food served a purpose by keeping me awake when I wanted to work, but now food was a problem. The size of my body interfered with things I wanted to do, like sit in a restaurant booth and fit in a public bathroom stall. I couldn't reach my feet, because my belly got in the way, so I had to ask my husband to put my shoes on me each morning. The extra weight I lugged around made it impossible to get up from the couch and even roll over in bed without struggling. And the embarrassment I felt about my appearance made me stop wearing shorts and swimsuits. Although I loved swimming, I no longer went in the water.

One morning, I hit rock bottom. There wasn't one specific thing that made me feel fed up with myself. I was just tired of not being able to do things I wanted to do. I stood in the kitchen, getting ready to make a high-calorie breakfast, when something just snapped inside of me. I blurted out, "Enough." Then I said it again with firmness and conviction: "Enough!" At that moment, my why changed. I no longer wanted to lose weight to please the people around me. I wanted to lose weight so I could do all the things I couldn't do as an obese person. The change in my why made all the difference in the world.

My new why switched my focus from negative to positive. Instead of running away from obesity because other people told me I should not be overweight, I was running toward all things I wanted to do: tie my shoes, fit in a restaurant booth, wear a seat belt. Instead of weight loss feeling oppressive, it felt liberating. I was filled with hope and energy for change. I was going somewhere. I had a new strength, and the next time I faced a bag of chocolate chip cookies, I was able to turn away.

Dieting

With a new why to support my actions, I started my diet. This time, I joined Weight Watchers and used the Weight Watchers app on my phone. I had been too proud to ask another human being for help with my weight loss. I didn't want to admit to myself or anyone else that I lacked the self-discipline to lose weight on my own, and the Weight Watchers app allowed me to get help anonymously.

The app suggested that as my first goal, I should work to lose 5 percent of my body weight. That would be 17 pounds, which seemed doable. The app also recommended losing 1 to 2 pounds per week. I did the math. In one year at that rate, I could lose 52 to 104 pounds. That was exciting. All I had to do was stick with the plan for a year. I also started to understand that my diet would not start and stop. I was beginning a lifestyle change that would continue for as long as I lived.

I learned a lot about myself from the Weight Watchers app. Each day, I logged my food and weight, and every time I lost another five pounds, a gold star appeared on the app's weight loss graph. I felt encouraged when I saw the downward slope of my weight loss, and I loved having the little stars appear every two weeks or so when I lost another five pounds. It was as if someone was saying, "Good job!" I felt supported and celebrated, and "Woohoo!" became a regular part of my vocabulary. I began to develop confidence that I had what it takes to lose weight. I learned that I do well when I break big goals into small goals, and that the goals that motivate me most are challenging but also realistic. I also thrive with daily accountability and frequent, but not too frequent, successes. I suspect the same is true for most people in all types of journeys.

While Weight Watchers promotes sound nutrition, I (at first) did not focus on nutrition. Instead, I just counted points without worrying about the types of foods making up those points. Since I loved carbs, I ate almost all of my points as carbs. I made gallons of fresh fruit chunks and ate them like popcorn in the evenings. But mostly, I used my points to consume sweets—cookies, cake, and candy bars. Often, I hit my point limit at breakfast by eating pancakes and doughnuts. Then I wouldn't eat for the rest of the day. The point system worked, and I lost 66 pounds over a nine-month period, a healthy average of 1 to 2 pounds per week. I was still obese, but I felt pretty slim at 269 pounds. However, the way I'd chosen to implement the Weight Watcher program was neither sustainable nor healthy.

Walking

My husband was concerned about my health and had been nagging me for years to exercise. I had no idea how to exercise as an obese person. It seemed impossible. At 335 pounds, I worried that I'd have a heart attack if I did anything physical. I also feared that I'd have joint injury from the impact of movement under so much weight. Walking seemed out of the question. The only place I walked was in the grocery store while holding onto a shopping cart for support. So every time Brian suggested that I exercise, I'd make some excuse and decline.

But after I lost 66 pounds, that changed. One evening, Brian said, "Come on, we're going for a walk." They were the same words

I had heard him say a million times before, but this time, I thought about it. Even though I was still obese, I felt stronger at 269 pounds. Maybe I could go for a walk. To my surprise, I said OK. I stood at the back door, terrified. *Why did I agree to do this? What was I thinking?* I grabbed Brian's arm and took a step. I had no idea that it would be the first step of a journey that would take me to the Age Group Triathlon World Championship. I was just hoping to get to the end of the driveway and back.

I walked down the driveway, turned the corner, and headed toward our neighbors' house. I made it to their driveway. Woohoo! I did it! Then I walked home. The entire walk was probably the length of a football field. I was utterly exhausted but felt on top of the world. After being inactive for years, I had exercised. I collapsed on the couch with a smile and a feeling of deep satisfaction.

The next day, we walked past our neighbors' house to the next neighbors' driveway before turning around. And the day after that, we walked to the third driveway. As the distance got farther, I had to take rest stops, but we kept going. Pretty soon, I could walk all the way around the block. That was a huge milestone. And then we walked an entire mile—another milestone. I never imagined I would ever walk a mile. I was pumped.

I discovered a wonderful app called Run Keeper and started logging the distance I walked each day. As with the Weight Watchers graph, I loved seeing the data as I logged the miles. Each day, I sent my sons, who were living in Georgia and Kentucky, a text like this one: "Walked 1.3 miles today! Woohoo!" They were so supportive. I'd get a return message that said, "Great job, Mom!" or "I'm proud of you!" I found their support so encouraging. Even today, I share my workouts with my sons, and I love when they say something encouraging after a hard bike ride or run.

Five Kilometers

One evening, after Brian and I had been walking for a few months, we left the house and started walking due east. We planned to walk a mile, the most I had ever walked, but instead of turning around at the half-mile point, I suggested we keep going east. We walked east for a total of one and a half miles. The only way to get home was to turn around and walk another one and a half miles—a total of three miles, or just short of five kilometers.

The last half mile of walking home was difficult. I wondered if I had made a terrible mistake. My feet hurt, and I had trouble concentrating. I asked my husband not to talk to me and just focused on keeping my legs moving. I told myself over and over to just make it to the next driveway. One by one, the driveways slid behind us. When we reached our driveway, I was over-the-moon proud. My heart had been pounding from exertion, but now it swelled with pride. *I did it!* I immediately texted my sons, "I just walked a 5k!!!!!!" Then I begged for a foot massage (which I got) and went to bed exhausted and happy.

While I didn't mention it to Brian at the time, I'd hoped to walk three miles for a reason. Our younger son, Andy, had been urging me to walk with him in a 5K event. Each time he brought it up, I told him he was crazy, but I made that my secret goal. I didn't really care about participating in an organized 5K with lots of people. But I thought walking in a 5K with Andy would be a great mother-son experience, and I wanted to see how far I could go.

Endurance Sports

After walking five kilometers in my neighborhood with Brian, I knew I could cover the distance. But I developed new hesitations. The next time Andy asked me to a 5K, I told him that 5Ks were for fit people, not obese people like me. He assured me that 5K events were designed for anyone, not just runners, and with some apprehension, I finally agreed to participate in a 5K event.

A few days later, Andy called to tell me he had found the perfect 5K for us. It was close to home, and the course was pretty flat. Then he told me the name of the race: the Krispy Kreme Challenge. I laughed when I heard the name—and even more when I learned about the race's unique twist. At the halfway point, each participant would be given a dozen doughnuts to eat. I envisioned everyone at the race seeing my obese body and assuming I had come just for the doughnuts. I laughed to myself when I realized that in addition to the challenge of walking a 5K, I would also be tempted to eat a dozen doughnuts. Too funny!

It never occurred to me to train competitively for the Krispy Kreme Challenge. I wasn't interested in going fast; I just wanted to finish. I kept walking in the evenings with Brian and made sure we walked five kilometers from time to time. If I could do five kilometers in my neighborhood, I figured I should be able to cross the finish line at the Krispy Kreme Challenge.

The week before the race, I was terrified—I mean, simply *terrified*. I had never witnessed a 5K, and I assumed everyone there would be fit and athletic. I didn't seem to belong in that group. My son again assured me that endurance sports are different from other sports. He explained there would be fast runners, but there would also be slow walkers and even people pushing strollers. He told me that everyone would be supportive and that the goal for most people was to finish, not to go fast. He added that people would be too worried about their own walk or run to be looking at me.

Even so, I was concerned. I didn't want my slowness to inconvenience anyone, and I was worried that the race sponsors and volunteers would have to wait around for me to finish. Based on the five-kilometer walks I had done at home, I calculated that it would take me close to an hour and a half to finish the race. I called the race coordinator, told her how long I thought I'd be on the course, and asked if the Krispy Kreme Challenge was an appropriate event for me. She assured me that even if I were far behind the last person, they would still be cleaning up, and no one would be inconvenienced. With that assurance, I gave Andy the go-ahead to register us for the race.

I wasn't sure what to wear for the Krispy Kreme Challenge. At home, I walked in regular street clothes, but that didn't seem appropriate for a 5K event. My weight was down, but I was still too big to fit into sizes offered by athletic brands at the time. I finally decided to wear stretch pants, a Life Is Good T-shirt (size XXXL), and a visor in case it was sunny. I felt strange—like an imposter—purchasing clothes designed for runners. I thought people might see me and wonder what the obese person was doing in sporty clothes. But at the same time, I felt excited to have new clothes for the big event.

The morning of the race, I could not keep my emotions under control. I was absolutely terrified. But more than that, I was excited and giggled like a schoolgirl. I couldn't believe I was wearing a race bib with a number on it—646. The whole thing seemed unreal. We took photos to mark the occasion, and I lined up with my son and husband at the very rear of all the runners and walkers, behind those pushing strollers. The announcer said, "Go," and as everyone moved forward, I did, too. Oh, my gosh! I was walking in an official 5K! I couldn't believe it, and as we crossed the start line, I teared up. My son ran ahead as we officially started, planning to double back and walk with my husband and me after finishing his run.

The course was an "out and back." That meant we would go to a turnaround point halfway through the route and then double back to the finish line. The first mile and a half flew by, and I felt pretty good. This walk was just like the five-kilometer walks at home, except lots of other people were walking too, which made it fun. The fast runners who had already passed the turnaround ran by us, going in the opposite direction. I cheered for each one running by us. A few said encouraging things to me, too: "Good job!" "You've got this!" Their kindness touched me and filled me with pride. We passed our son, who also was running back, and he cheered loudly for me, which made my heart sing.

As we approached the turnaround, I saw boxes of Krispy Kreme doughnuts sitting on a big white table. Volunteers were passing them out, and many participants had stopped walking or running to sit on the grass and eat doughnuts, as though they were enjoying a picnic. I knew everyone would see the obese person and figure I'd stop for doughnuts, but I wasn't even tempted. Doughnuts were something the old Sue would have liked. The new Sue just wanted to cross the finish line without dying.

Just beyond the table of doughnuts, another table was covered with little paper cups full of water. Volunteers handed them out to the runners as they passed. I didn't know what to do. I assumed the water was for the runners. I was just a walker. It seemed rude for me to take a cup of water that was meant for the athletes, not for obese participants like me. It wasn't just that I didn't need water. In my head, I didn't deserve water. I wasn't doing anything notable. I wasn't an athlete. So I walked past the table. But as I did, one of the volunteers ran out from behind the table and handed *me* a cup of water! That moment changed my life. That little cup of water and her recognition of my effort made me *feel* like an athlete. In my head, I was competing in the Boston Marathon, where volunteers supported me with water along the way. For the first time ever, I got a glimpse of what it feels like to be an athlete—and I loved that feeling.

The next one and a half miles of walking were excruciating. I must have gotten carried away and walked faster than normal during the first half. My heart raced. I couldn't talk. I couldn't focus. Everything hurt. My son had finished his race and circled back to join us. Hearing my husband and son talking to each other was totally distracting. I needed every bit of my focus to keep my feet moving. I gasped, "Please don't talk," and focused on my feet. That strategy worked, and to this day, when running is tough at the end of a race, I tune out everything and will my feet to not slow down.

As I approached the finish line, I was dead last, but I didn't care. I was filled with excitement. I was about to complete my first 5K. I was happy beyond belief as I approached the finish line, and the announcer said, "And here comes Sue Reynolds! This is her first 5K!" To my amazement, everyone who was still there stopped what they were doing and started clapping and cheering. At the halfway point, I had felt like I was running in the Boston Marathon. Now I felt like I had won the Boston Marathon. The moment was joyous, and I felt the deep satisfaction that comes with completing a challenging task. I completed the Krispy Kreme Challenge in one hour and fifteen minutes—an average pace of twenty-four minutes and eight seconds per mile, which is slow as molasses. But to this day, that is the hardest event I have ever completed, and it is the event of which I am proudest.

During the Krispy Kreme Challenge, I was bitten by the endurance-sports bug. I loved witnessing the athletes' joy as they waited for the race to start. I loved how some participants were elite runners, while others were recreational runners and some, like me, were struggling just to finish. I loved that we all were on the same course and that everyone supported each other. The elites cheered for me. I cheered for the elites. And most surprising, I discovered that I loved pushing my body to its limits.

Running

During the three months after walking in the Krispy Kreme Challenge, I struggled to stay within my Weight Watchers point goals. I had trouble sustaining the physical effort when I ate all my points at breakfast and then limited my food intake for the rest of the day, so I started eating throughout the day. Thankfully, my daily walks and participation in additional 5K events kept me from gaining weight, and I hovered between 260 and 270 pounds.

As I walked, my fitness continued to increase, and I found myself wondering if I could run. I wasn't sure if my body could support my weight, but I wanted to try. Secretly, I tried running a few steps— about ten feet in total. The sensation of running seemed foreign and awkward. I felt a little silly to be attempting a run when I weighed around 265 pounds. To be honest, I'm not sure I was actually running, but my arms were bent and moving relatively fast, so I called it running. With my extra weight, I couldn't lean forward as runners do, so I compensated by taking tiny steps with a quick cadence. I made the ten feet, and then fifteen, and then fifty. I started to feel excited. I was running.

I learned about a free app called Run 5k, an online interval training program, and decided to try it. Basically, Run 5k has you do a combination of walking and running three times a week with rest days in between. On the first day, you jog for forty-five seconds.

That felt doable to me. Then the jog time increases slowly over the weeks, and two months later, you're running an entire five kilometers. The slow progression keeps you from getting injured. I liked that approach.

I weighed 267 pounds when I started the Run 5k program. On the first day, I turned on the app and heard a pleasant voice say, "Walk." I walked for five minutes. That was the warm-up. Then the voice said, "Run!" I knew the jog would only be for forty-five seconds and would be followed by a longer walk period. I started running. For the next twenty-four minutes, I alternated between walking and jogging ten times, then walked an additional five minutes to cool down. Each week, the jog time increased, and after eight weeks, I could actually run for thirty minutes.

The program's slow progression from walking to running resulted in no injury—until I went rogue during the last week of the program and did more than the voice told me to do. I was having a good day and decided to keep running after the voice said to walk for the cooldown. Throwing common sense aside, I also decided to run fast rather than jog. The next day, I noticed a little ache in my right hip. It was not a sharp pain, just a little niggle. Today I would simply train through that type of pain, but that was the first time I had ever felt pain from exercise, and I freaked out. I was scared I had injured myself for life. I didn't know what to do.

I decided to see my doctor, an internist with a reputation for being very conservative. I told him about my weight loss, running, and the pain I had in my right hip. He thought for a long time. Finally, he told me to stop running until I weighed 220 pounds. I was devastated but followed his advice. Looking back, I wish I had gone to a sports doctor who had experience with runners and a mission of helping people return from injury to exercise. I think I would have gotten different advice. But at the time, I didn't think of myself as an athlete, and it never occurred to me that I could go to a sports doctor. I followed the internist's advice and stopped running.

It was difficult to keep my resolve at this point in my journey. I continued to walk around the neighborhood but didn't enter any more 5K events. Staying within my Weight Watchers points became even more challenging, and as the winter months passed, with all of the holiday customs that involved food, my willpower collapsed. Eating with abandon became more and more frequent, and I started failing to log. As I put on weight, I became concerned that this was becoming one more failed attempt at weight loss.

Chapter 3

RESET

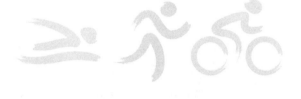

I had lot of experience with the path I seemed to be on: lose lots of weight, then gain it all back. With a new why and after losing 66 pounds, I'd had high hopes that this time would be different, but it seemed like it wasn't. I'd stop on the way home from work at my favorite bakery, purchase a dozen huge cookies, and then consume them on the drive home; go to restaurants that had large dessert buffets, and just happen to stroll past Blu Boy Chocolate Store where I'd stop in to purchase chocolates and macarons. Within nine months, I regained almost half of the 66 pounds I had lost, and my weight climbed back to 304 pounds.

I started feeling hopeless again. Dieting obviously wasn't working for me. It seemed the only route to weight loss for someone like me was surgery, but I didn't feel that was the right option for me. Once again, I started believing that I would just be heavy all my life. At the same time, however, my new why kept nagging at me. I couldn't stop thinking about all the things I couldn't do because of my size and about my goal to run, rather than walk, in a 5K event. I seemed to be stuck between two loves: eating sweets and doing all the things I wanted to do but couldn't because of my size.

Then a friend invited me to join a three-month exercise program she had been doing in a small fitness studio in our town. The program's website showed before-and-after photos of people who had lost over a hundred pounds. Those photos gave me hope and made me wonder if I should enroll in the program, but signing up for the class would mean admitting I couldn't do it on my own. Finally, I told myself that after multiple attempts over many years, I had not been successful at losing weight on my own. I needed help. I needed community. I swallowed my pride and signed up for the program.

I literally cringed when I learned the name of the program: Meltdown Bootcamp. That sounded intimidating. I pictured myself doing push-ups with a trainer in my face, screaming at me to do one more. Maybe I was crazy to even think about doing that program. I questioned my friend repeatedly. I wanted to make sure that someone weighing more than three hundred pounds could survive a boot camp. My friend assured me that other obese people would be part of the program. She added that most of the instructors had been my size at one point in their lives. I wasn't so sure, but I agreed to go.

My friend and I planned to go together to the first class, but as I drove into the parking lot, I received a text from her saying she would not be able to come. I felt panic-stricken. I had never been to a gym before. I didn't know anyone there. I thought about turning the car around and driving home. But instead, I pulled into a parking spot and stopped, debating what to do. All my life, I had chosen to let my actions be controlled by fear or pride instead of by my desire to be healthy. I was twenty feet from the front door. All I had to do was walk through that door. I got out of the car and walked up to the building.

The front door was glass, and I could see inside. Mats lay on the floor in what appeared to be a circle with dumbbells and balls sitting next to them. People were standing around and chatting. I stopped abruptly in front of the door, terrified and unsure of what to do next. Then I did something I've repeated often throughout my journey. I held my hands in front of me palms up, like two trays on a balance scale. In my left hand, I imagined my fear and pride—the things that made me want to make a poor choice. In the other hand, I imagined all the things I wanted to be able to do—sit in a restaurant booth, use a regular-size restroom stall, run in a 5K. Then I rocked my hands up and down slightly, the way people do when they are trying to make a decision. A second later, I said out loud with firmness, "Go away, pride! Go away, fear!" Then I made myself walk through the door.

Once inside, I just stood. I had no idea what to do. Thankfully, a woman came up and asked if I wanted to be her partner for the class. I felt so grateful for her kindness, without which I might have run back out the door. The class involved rotating from mat to mat. A card at each mat told you what to do. When the instructor yelled, "Go!" you'd begin the exercise. A little while later, she'd yell, "Stop!" and you'd rotate to the next station.

My first problem was that, at 304 pounds, I could not do *any* of the things that were written on the cards. I could not do a push-up. I had never heard of a mountain climber. Luckily, my friend had explained that if I couldn't do something, I should raise my hand and ask for an alternative exercise. The first station was push-ups. I raised my hand. The instructor, Maria, was wonderful. She quickly came and told me to do push-ups against the wall instead of the floor. That was still challenging for a person my size, but it was doable. At the second station, I raised my hand, and again at the third and fourth stations. Finally, Maria just started coming over to me with each rotation to give me an alternative.

My second problem was that I couldn't get up from the floor quickly enough to move to the next station before Maria shouted, "Go!" Getting off the floor meant I had to get on my hands and knees, then progress to hands and feet, and then hopefully struggle to a stand. It just took too long, so I ended up crawling on my hands and knees from station to station, with my pride screaming at me to run out the door. As I crawled, I said to myself over and over, *Go away, pride. Go away, pride. Go away, pride!*

The station I feared the most was Jacob's ladder. It was a ladder with rungs that moved downward as you climbed. For safety reasons, you put on a belt that is tethered to the ladder. If you fall, the rotating rungs stop moving. My heart stopped when I saw the belt. I was sure it wouldn't fit around my wide belly. So embarrassing! *Go away, pride.* I was doubly sure I would fall off the moving ladder. *Go away, fear.* As I moved around the stations, closer and closer to Jacob's ladder, my dread grew. Finally, I was standing in front of the ladder. As I put on the belt, I wondered who the heck Jacob was. I decided he was a sick sadist who took great joy in seeing others suffer as they tried to climb the ladder's rungs. Thankfully, the belt fit—a huge relief. I started up the ladder—one step, then another. The rungs started to move downward under my feet as I climbed. I was doing it. Maria had been watching. She yelled loudly across the room in front of everyone, "Good job, Sue!" I felt like a little kid just bursting with pride.

After class, I sat in the parking lot and cried—partly from exhaustion, but mainly happy tears full of joy. I did it! I survived the class, and I had climbed Jacob's ladder! I was soaking wet with perspiration. For the first time in decades, it wasn't perspiration from the heat. It was sweat from exertion. I loved every drop, savoring the sensation of accomplishment.

The Bootcamp program included exercise classes twice a week, but I couldn't handle that in the beginning. I'd go to class on Mondays and then be tired for the next four days. After the first few weeks, it became easier, and I started going to class on Mondays and Thursdays. I always tried to go to class when Maria was teaching. Her attention and kind words inspired me.

After each exercise class and any other time I exercised on my own, I logged my exercise on a form provided by the Meltdown Bootcamp. At the end of the week, I sent the log to Bill, the exercise coach assigned to me. Each week, he'd assign a letter grade to my effort, based on how many hours I logged. I quickly learned to log my hours a week in advance and then follow the plan I'd created to earn an A. I liked having a weekly plan to follow, and I liked seeing the As that appeared on my record. In addition to reviewing our logs, Bill sometimes attended the exercise classes. He got in front of people like a drill sergeant and yelled, "One more rep! Give me one more rep!" Luckily, he never did that to me. I suspect he tailored his coaching style for each individual person. He knew that instead of inspiring me, that approach would crush me.

In addition to the exercise program, Meltdown Bootcamp also had a nutrition program. They described it as a whole-foods, low-sugar program with carb cycling. Each day, I ate five assigned meals of proteins, healthy carbs, fats, and vegetables. I was given a list of foods that were approved for each food group, along with the quantity that made up a serving. Carbs had to be healthy carbs, like oatmeal and brown rice, not the sweet carbs (like cookies and candy) that I enjoyed eating. At the beginning of the week, we received instructions about which food groups to eat for each meal. On some days, we ate no carbs, while other days were heavy carbs. While not all agree, some nutrition consultants believe that this type of carb rotation contributes to weight loss. Meals had to be at least three hours apart, and every two weeks, the plan changed slightly. I also had to drink 120 ounces of water every day. It seemed like I was putting food or water into my mouth every minute. Instead of telling myself not to eat, I had to remind myself to eat. I was surprised that my stomach never felt hungry—not even once. And the balance provided by this meal plan made a huge difference for me: rather than eating all my points in sweets early in the day, I now had a plan geared toward nutrition throughout the day.

The Bootcamp nutrition plan included a weekly cheat day, which I loved. On those days, I could eat whatever I wanted. During exercise class, we loved to talk about the wonderful foods we planned to eat on cheat day. For many, it was pizza and beer. For me, it was waffles smothered with maple syrup. At first, I went hog wild with cheat days and would often consume three or four thousand calories. But I quickly realized I was undoing all the good I had done in the previous week. Determined to keep making progress, I switched to cheat meals rather than cheat days. It was nice to have those fun foods once in a while, but after the first three weeks in the program, I stopped craving foods that were not on the approved list and started craving foods that nourished my body and gave me energy.

Like the exercise program, Bootcamp also had an accountability system for my eating. Every evening, I'd send my nutrition coach, Barb, an email that listed the foods I had eaten that day and quantities. A short while later, she'd send a return email to say, "Good job!" or let me know where I had messed up. After a while, Barb and

I started sharing little bits about how our days went. She was like a pen pal.

Barb always looked for the positive. When I ate a half gallon of chocolate-dusted almonds in one sitting, Barb complimented me for throwing the remaining half away. That accountability and support had been missing in my failed diets. I'd like to think I could have lost weight without this level of accountability, but the reality is that I was not successful on my own. I needed support and community.

My exercise and nutrition coaches monitored the degree to which I implemented Bootcamp's process, but the founder and director of Bootcamp, Adam, monitored the outcome. At the start of Bootcamp, we each had to stand privately on a scale before Adam while he recorded our weight on a spreadsheet. When it was my turn, I set my resolve. *Go away, pride.* The scale read 304. I waited for Adam to say something about my massive weight, but he just told me how happy he was that I was there. Then, every two weeks, we each stood before Adam again as he updated our weight.

On the second weigh-in, the pressure was on. I had followed the exercise program and nutrition perfectly, and my scale at home indicated a weight loss, but I had no idea what Adam's scale would say. When the digital numbers popped on the scale, Adam simply said, "Niiiiice!" I learned to love that one-syllable word and hoped I would hear it every two weeks when I weighed in. Even after Bootcamp ended and I was down to 235 pounds, I continued to weigh in with Adam every two weeks for years. Meltdown Bootcamp, with its encouragement and accountability, was my lifeline.

One of the biggest lessons I learned from Bootcamp was to be coachable. At the start of Bootcamp, I questioned everything. Why didn't we have carbs on some days? Why weren't we allowed to have dairy products? Why couldn't we drink diet pop? Finally, Adam told me firmly to let him do the thinking and to just do what he told me to do. End of discussion.

To be honest, that made me a little mad. I didn't like being told to not think. Childishly, I decided to prove that Adam's program didn't work. My plan was to do exactly what he said, and then at the end of Bootcamp, my lack of weight loss would make it obvious that his program was flawed. I followed his plan to the letter every day. At the end of three months, I had lost thirty pounds. His program worked.

I was pleased with far more than the weight loss. I had learned so much about exercise, nutrition, and accountability. I learned to let go of control and put myself into the hands of a trusted coach. Most of all, I had confidence that I had the knowledge and strength to continue my weight loss journey on my own after the three-month Bootcamp ended.

My first step after Bootcamp was to find a means to continue logging my food that included food types and quantities, rather than points. I found an easy-to-use free app called My Fitness Pal, which not only allowed me to log my food and weight each day, but also provided a nice daily report about the food groups I had eaten that day. I started developing my own food plans, using what I had learned in Bootcamp. I entered my food plans into My Fitness Pal ahead of time, instead of logging my foods after I ate them. Then during the day, I simply followed the plan I had created by eating the foods that were already in my log. That helped me stay on track.

Each evening before going to bed, I reviewed My Fitness Pal. On days that I followed my plan perfectly, I'd tell myself, *Good job!* Then each morning, I'd weigh myself and enter my weight into My Fitness Pal. Every time I dropped an additional five pounds, I'd say, *Woohoo!* when I saw the weight on the scale. After years of failed attempts at losing weight, I finally found a system that was highly sustainable for me. I've been logging my food and taking my weight daily, with a few lapses, ever since.

My weight loss journey wasn't perfect. I made mistakes along the way, but I learned from them. On a weeklong vacation, I decided to do a cheat *week* instead of a cheat day, figuring that I'd get right back on track when I returned home. That was a disaster. I quickly learned that if I cheat for more than two days, it is incredibly difficult (but not impossible) for me to get back on track. That cheat week turned into a cheat month before I successfully restarted. I also learned that after slipping, I only needed enough willpower to turn away from fun food for two days. After that, it became easier to say no to the temptation, because a healthy eating pattern had resumed. It wasn't a perfect journey, but I made progress.

I discovered mental strategies that worked for me, too. For example, I told myself I needed to set boundaries with food, just as I set boundaries with people. Boundaries with people keep me from engaging in unhealthy relationships. Boundaries with food keep me from engaging in unhealthy eating. At times, I even talked to my food. When facing cookies and candy, I'd say firmly, "You are not going to hurt me. I have boundaries." Then I'd turn away.

Another mental strategy was to observe the behavior of healthy people and then imitate those behaviors. This is a strategy I've used often in my life to help me develop the traits of people I admire. In this case, I was not yet at a healthy body weight, but there was no reason why I couldn't act like a healthy person. The healthiest person I knew was my daughter-in-law Laura. She was fit and worked hard to take care of her physical well-being. When we were together, I watched what she ate. In restaurants, I tried to order after she did.

When it was my turn, I asked for whatever Laura had ordered. I did the same thing with exercise, except in that case, I went to the YMCA, observed fit people, and tried to copy their routines.

One of my favorite mental strategies was to pretend that healthy foods were fun foods. I cut my apples into thin slices and pretended they were potato chips. I loved the sense of munching as one slice after another went into my mouth. I added extracts and sweetener to plain Greek yogurt and imagined it was lemon meringue pie or an orange Creamsicle. A tablespoon of almond butter mixed with sweetener became a Reese's Peanut Butter Cup.

I also learned to control my environment. I went to the grocery store frequently so there wouldn't be a lot of food in the house. I volunteered to bring a dish to parties to ensure there was something healthy I could eat. After family get-togethers, I sent food home with people, so I wouldn't eat it all as soon as they left. People often tell me that I must have a lot of willpower to have lost two hundred pounds. I don't think that's the case. I just became pretty good at controlling my environment to eliminate the temptation.

Slowly, the pounds continued to come off at a healthy 1 to 2 pounds per week. After being on my own for six months following Bootcamp, I crossed the 100-pounds-lost line. On the morning the scale read 235 pounds, I couldn't believe it. After so many failed diets, I never imagined I would lose 100 pounds. I shared the news with my husband and then sent a text to my sons. My heart swelled as they all told me how proud they were of me. And I felt excited about the future. I knew I had a sustainable plan that would take me through the next 100 pounds, as well as the strength to stick with it. I couldn't wait to move forward and start running again.

TRIATHLON SEASON 1

CROSSING THE START LINE

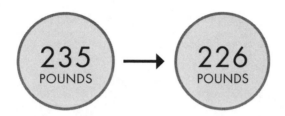

235 POUNDS → 226 POUNDS

Chapter 4

FIRST TRIATHLON

A t 235 pounds, I wasn't quite at the weight where my doctor wanted me to be before I started running again, but I was close enough. I started out nice and easy, once again using the Run 5k app to build my run distance. This time, I didn't do more than the voice told me to do, and I stayed injury free.

In addition to running, I enrolled in a water aerobics class to give my exercise some variety. I purchased a swimsuit with an attached skirt that hung to my knees and covered much of my healthier but still obese body. I loved water aerobics. It was the perfect physical activity for an obese person. Moving through the water gave my heart a workout and helped with flexibility, without putting strain on my joints. After one class, I decided to see if I could swim at my large size. I kicked a length with a kickboard. So far, so good. Then I tried a length of breaststroke and made it without drowning.

Swimming two to four lengths after water aerobics class became part of my routine.

And then it occurred to me: if I added cycling, I could do a triathlon. I don't know what made me think of that. I didn't know anyone who had ever done a triathlon. I had never even seen a triathlon. I vaguely remembered feeling impressed twenty years earlier when someone told me that her husband had completed a triathlon in Hawaii. Maybe I could do a triathlon. Maybe I could be a triathlete. I started researching triathlon online and discovered the shorter sprint triathlon. I could already run the sprint's 5K. I could swim four lengths in a pool and thought I could build that to the 30 lengths I'd need to equal the sprint's half-mile swim distance. But I hadn't ridden a bike in forty years.

In reality, I didn't think I would ever actually do a triathlon, but that became my secret daydream, as walking a 5K had been a year earlier. When I was exercising, I imagined that I was training for a triathlon. I increased my swim distance each week and over time worked toward 0.5 miles. I joined a spin class and noted how many miles I rode in class, hoping to come close to the sprint's 12.4-mile bike segment. Again, I wasn't trying to prepare for a triathlon. I just liked how the secret daydream gave purpose to my exercise. But with time, I could swim, cycle, and run the distance that sprint triathletes raced. The question was whether I could do all three consecutively.

As I researched triathlons online, I stumbled across an indoor triathlon that was being sponsored by the swim club at Indiana University near my home in a couple of months. Maybe I could use that indoor triathlon as a test. I would have to swim six hundred meters in a pool, ride eight miles on a spin bike, and then run three miles around an indoor track. Between events, I could go into the locker room to change clothes, eat a snack, or rest for as long as I liked.

I couldn't imagine doing a triathlon. That seemed preposterous for a sixty-year-old woman who had been sitting on a couch for almost fifty years. But out of curiosity, I sent an email to the college student who was in charge of the event. I explained that it would take me a long time to finish and asked what she thought. "We'll put you in the first wave," she cheerfully replied. "You'll have plenty of time." I wasn't so sure, but in a moment of insanity, I registered for the event.

The morning of the race was crazy. I had purchased a new, skirtless swimsuit for the event and felt self-conscious when a volunteer wrote my race number on my upper arms and thighs with a black magic marker. When it was time for my wave, they told us to each jump in the water and get into a lane by ourselves. I whispered to the college student who was timing me, "I hope you brought a book. It's going to take me quite a while to swim twenty-four lengths of the pool." Then I jumped in and held on to the side of the pool as I waited for the start of my wave. I could feel my heart pounding in my chest, and my eyes misted slightly as I thought about how far I had come since that first walk to the mailbox.

The air horn sounded, and I pushed off the wall. I still couldn't swim freestyle well, so I alternated breaststroke with freestyle. My student timer started cheering for me every time I came up to breathe in the breaststroke. When I climbed out of the water, she called me a rock star. I went to the locker room with a huge smile on my face, had a long rest, and then found the spin bikes where I rode for eight miles. After another long rest, I made twenty-four trips around the indoor track. Every time I came around to the start/finish line, the college kids cheered: "Go, Sue! You've got this, Sue!" Their enthusiasm carried me around and around until all three miles had been run. My husband was so excited that he ran down the track to give me a big hug—before I crossed the finish line! After his hug, I ran across the line. I was exhausted but deeply satisfied. I did it! I was a triathlete!

A few days later, filled with newfound confidence, I purchased a bike. It was an entry-level road bike with handlebars that curved down. I told the fellow at the bike shop that I hadn't ridden a bike in forty years and was worried I'd scratch the bike during the test ride if I fell. He assured me that riding would come back to me—and it did. As I rode down a nearby bike path and felt the wind blow across my face, I felt like a bird flying through the air. I loved that feeling. Glorious! I purchased the bike and began riding outside, enjoying every mile.

It occurred to me that my daydream about doing a triathlon wasn't a daydream anymore. I started reading everything I could find on triathlon. I discovered that triathlons are for all kinds of people. You don't have to be a good athlete or fast competitor. Many people do triathlons slowly with the goal of finishing. You don't even have to be a good swimmer. There are boats all along the swim course, and you're allowed to hold on to a boat while resting, as long as you don't make forward progress. Some people do backstroke, breaststroke, or even dog paddle during the swim. And finally, you don't have to have good equipment. You just need a swimsuit, running shoes, and a bike—any old bike.

With this knowledge, I signed up for my first outdoor triathlon, a sprint triathlon in Indianapolis that would be held in July, only four months away. To prepare, I just continued the exercise I had done in the past, alternating swim, bike, and run each day—except it wasn't exercising anymore. Now it was training. I was training for my first outdoor triathlon with an open-water swim.

As race day approached, I needed to figure out what to wear. From my research, I knew most people wore a special triathlon outfit called a "tri kit." Basically, a tri kit is a skintight tank top connected to skintight shorts. But at 226 pounds, I had too many jiggly parts to feel comfortable running in anything that was skintight, and while many manufacturers make tri kits in plus sizes today, they did not have tri kits for larger women a few years ago. I finally decided to wear my swimsuit and put on capri-length running pants and a T-shirt over it after I finished the swim. I also brought a cover-up, so my body would be hidden until the very start of the race.

But I couldn't figure out how to get into a bra after the swim. As a large woman, my chest would do considerable bouncing if it wasn't somehow contained (blush!). I knew there was something called a sports bra, but I had no idea what that was. The only person I knew who might know was Megan, the woman who had taught my spin class. With much embarrassment, I asked Megan if she knew what a sports bra was. She smiled and said, "Yes! I have one on right now!" She explained that many women wear sports bras under their bathing suits or tri kits in triathlons, so that's what I did. I was a little embarrassed that my bra straps showed under my suit, but then I remembered Brandi Chastain ripping off her shirt after Team USA won the Women's Soccer World Cup Championship in 1999. I figured if she could run around in her sports bra, I could let mine show a little bit.

My weight had been fluctuating since the preceding Christmas. On New Year's Day, I weighed 242 pounds. Evidently, I had not quite mastered the willpower that would come later in my journey. But I had learned that I could reset, and that's what I did. My weight went down to 216, only to increase again over the Fourth of July holiday. Holidays with all their wonderful foods were proving to be my downfall. On the morning of my first outdoor triathlon, my weight was down 109 pounds but still obese for someone with my height and body type.

At my first outdoor triathlon, I had never swum in a lake, other than to float around on a raft. I had never ridden my bike on a road with cars. I had never even seen a triathlon transition area. And I was still grossly overweight. I hadn't told anyone except my family what I was about to do. To be honest, I was a little afraid I would back out at the last moment. If I did, I didn't want anyone to know.

The day before the race, my husband and I drove to the hotel where we would spend the night. On the way, we stopped at a running shop, where race packets were being distributed. My first race packet! I eagerly opened the drawstring bag to see what was inside: a race bib, a race number to stick on my bike, a swim cap, a race T-shirt, a timing chip on a Velcro strap, a few gels, and some advertisements. As I went through the contents, I found my excitement starting to mount. This was really happening. I was about to do an outdoor triathlon.

After picking up my race packet, we drove the bike course in the car, and my excitement turned to fear. The hills were too steep. There were cars on the road. But when we got to the hotel, my emotions turned again to excitement as I rolled my bike through the hotel lobby. "Look at me," I wanted to shout. "I have a bike! I'm going to race tomorrow!" When I went to bed that night, my stomach was full of butterflies. I barely slept, thinking of all that was coming the next day.

The alarm went off at 4:00 a.m., and the butterflies were still there. I considered backing out but decided to postpone that decision until I got to the race. I quickly ate the breakfast I'd read triathletes were supposed to eat: a plain bagel, peanut butter, a banana, and lots of water. These foods were *not* part of my regular nutrition plan, and I savored every single bite. Then I got ready for the race.

Before leaving the hotel, I pinned my race bib to my T-shirt. Then I put my shirt into a gym bag along with my capris, bike helmet, shoes, socks, a beach towel, and other things I wanted to have in transition.

My husband and I arrived at the race venue at 6:00 a.m., two hours before the race was to start. Having never seen a triathlon before, I had no idea what to expect. We parked the car and walked a half mile to the transition area, a parking lot where participants would switch from swim to bike and then from bike to run. When we got there, I saw long sawhorses made out of galvanized pipe. Each sawhorse was about twenty feet long and four feet high. They were parallel to each other, with one end of each sawhorse touching the outside edge of the parking lot. A sign posted on the other end of each sawhorse listed a range of participant numbers, for example, 450–457.

A few participants were already there, and I could see that they were hanging their bikes by the front tip of the saddle on the crossbar of the metal sawhorses. They were also placing items they would need for the bike and run underneath their bike on a towel. I found a young man who had a fancy bike and looked accomplished. "This is my first triathlon," I said. "I don't know what I'm doing." His response was my first experience with the kindness of the triathlon community. He stopped what he was doing, showed me where to hang my bike, explained how to set up my transition area, and gave me a couple of tips.

I hung my bike by the seat and put everything I needed for the bike and run on a towel to one side of my front tire, which was touching the ground. I also laid on the towel many other things I didn't need: a second towel so I could dry off after the swim, a cooler with a sandwich and snacks, a hairbrush and hair tie, and a duffel bag with extra clothing. I wanted to be prepared for anything. I put my phone in the pocket of a run belt I planned to wear, so I could call my husband to come get me if I couldn't make the distance. Finally, I put some sugar cubes in a little box strapped to the front of my bike—just in case I needed extra energy.

After I set up my transition spot, it was time for "marking." A volunteer wrote my race number on my upper arms. My excitement started to surge. I had race numbers on my arms. Again I thought, *This is happening!* I attached the Velcro strip with my timing chip to my left ankle. Someone had told me to put it on my left ankle so it wouldn't hit my front derailleur, the part of the bike that shifts gears, when I pedaled.

The last step was to go to the restroom, where I discovered there was no toilet paper. I was thankful that several of the triathlon articles I read advised bringing toilet paper to events, and I had come prepared. I passed out handfuls of toilet paper to all the women in line.

Now I was ready for the start. In some triathlons, everyone starts at the same time. However, this triathlon was a time-trial start. Participants would enter the water one at a time with about two seconds between participants. That spreads out the swimmers and increases safety. When we registered, we stated our swimming ability, and the race organizer used that information to assign race numbers, so the faster swimmers would start first. I reported that I was slow.

A few minutes before 8:00 a.m., the announcer instructed us to get in line by number. Thankfully, we didn't have to be in strict numerical order, so I moved to the very back, where I would be around few swimmers. Once again, I felt panicky. I had never seen a triathlon start. I was hoping that by the time the hundreds of people ahead of me were in the water, I would know what was going on.

As I waited for my turn to start the swim, I focused on advice my younger son had given me a few days earlier. He had told me in a calm and peaceful voice, "Mom, this is no big deal. It's just a leisurely swim, followed by a relaxing bike ride, followed by an easy jog—just a nice day in the fresh air." I also thought about what my brother had told me about the safety of the course: "The race directors are not going to create a course that is dangerous. They want everyone to finish safely." Their reassuring words helped, but still, my heart was pounding.

It took about twenty minutes to get from the first swimmer to me. Right before my turn, I slipped out of my cover-up and handed it to my husband. Then I ran under the start arch and down the beach toward the water. I knew that all of my jiggly body parts were jiggling as I ran, and I told my pride to go away. Then I saw him. An official photographer was crouched at the side of the water, and as I ran into the water in my bathing suit with all my jiggly parts jiggling, he took my picture. Ugh. Silently, I screamed to myself, *Go away, pride.* Right before entering the water, I crossed a timing mat. The twenty minutes between the first starter and me would be subtracted from my time at the end.

As I started to swim, I panicked as I realized I couldn't see through the muddy water. It wasn't like swimming through the clear pool water, where I could follow a line on the bottom of the pool. The water was so muddy I couldn't even see my hands in front of me. I might as well have been swimming with my eyes closed! Then I remembered reading about sighting during triathlon swims, and every few strokes, I raised my head to make sure I was swimming straight to the turn buoy and to see where the other swimmers were. Since I was at the back of the swim, no one was trying to go fast.

When people bumped into me, they would lift their heads and say, "Sorry!" A few times, I swam breaststroke just so I could raise my head and look around. Little by little I started to relax and started enjoying the swim.

I learned to sense where other swimmers were by feeling the churning water as they kicked. By the time we got to the first yellow buoy, everyone spread out, and I could swim freestyle without worrying about running into people. I tried to work on form but mostly focused on conserving energy for the bike. I even swam a little without kicking to save my legs. After the last buoy, I swam toward shore until my hands hit sand, and then I stood and walked out of the lake. I found the pair of flip-flops I had hidden by the swim exit and slowly walked to the transition area, saving as much energy as I could.

I took my time in transition. I put on my capris and T-shirt over my bathing suit . . . sat down . . . put on my socks and shoes . . . drank some water . . . ate a sandwich . . . and even brushed my hair. Then, still trying to save energy, I slowly walked my bike out of transition. I now understand that the transition is part of the triathlon race, and triathletes try to race through transition, but I didn't understand it then. And even if I had understood, my goal was to finish, not to go fast. I was conserving every ounce of energy I had in hope of finishing all three events.

I loved, loved, loved the bike portion of the race. The course was hilly, and in the beginning, I was afraid of going fast on the downhills. Cautiously, I applied the brakes all the way down each hill. Then I had to work like crazy to get up the next hill. But at least I wasn't walking up the hills as I had feared. After a while, I discovered that if I rode as fast as possible down the hills (*go away, fear*), I could coast about two-thirds of the way up the next hill. By the time I finished, I flew up and down the hills. It was exhilarating.

My fears about riding with cars proved to be unfounded. One car passed me in the park, but at a super-slow speed. No problem. Once we left the park, we rode on a four-lane highway with cars. However, the race director had coned off the outside lane in each direction. Cars were using the outside lanes, and bikes were using the inside lanes. At each intersection, a police officer directed traffic. I never felt unsafe and appreciated all of the volunteers and police officers who yelled encouragement along the way. As I passed them, I shouted, "Thank you!" A couple of times, I just yelled "Wheeeeeee!" in pure joy as I sped past. I was having so much fun.

When I finished the bike segment and approached the transition area, I realized I didn't know where the dismount line was. I got off my bike way too soon and then had to run with my bike down the road to transition. Luckily, you don't have to actually be on your bike when you race. You just have to be touching it, so there was no penalty. Phew. I racked my bike and then slowly walked to the start of the run.

I knew the run would be challenging, and it was. It started with an incredibly steep uphill. I felt as if I was climbing the side of a mountain. Determined not to walk, I ran very, very slowly. I overheard one little boy on the sidelines say to his father, "Daddy, look! She's really slow." That made me laugh inside. I knew I was slow, but I was elated to be competing in my first triathlon.

When I drove the course the day before to scope out the challenge in front of me, I thought the route was uphill (slightly) on the way to the turnaround and then downhill on the way back. But as I was running, it seemed to be uphill both ways. I know that's not possible, but I swear I ran uphill for the entire three miles.

When I got to the turnaround, I again felt elated. I knew I was going to finish, and joy filled me. However, I still had a long way to go. When I was about a half mile from the finish line, I started passing participants who had already finished and were leaving. I was barely holding it together and was no longer confident about finishing. I focused on my cadence to keep from walking. *It doesn't matter that your body feels horrible,* I told myself. *Put the pain out of your mind. It is just pain. It does not matter. Do* not *slow your cadence.*

Then one of the finishers who was on his way home cheered for me as I ran by: "Way to go!" One by one, almost every person I passed yelled encouragement. "You've got this!" "Round the corner and down the hill!" "Looking strong!" One young man shouted, "Nice cadence!" I loved that he found something positive about my waddling shuffle. But my favorite cheer came from a woman who said, "Good job, runner!" No one had ever called me a runner before. Inside my exhausted body, I beamed with happiness.

With a quarter mile to go, a war occurred inside of me. My body screamed at my brain to stop its misery, while my brain screamed at my body to keep moving: *Stop. Keep going. Stop! Keep going!* For my brain to prevail, I needed to put every bit of my focus into maintaining my cadence, and the cheering people were making that challenging.

Every time I thanked a well-wisher, my legs slowed down. After a while, I didn't have enough gas in the tank to even say thank you. Even a head nod was too much effort. So I just ran down the road, one foot after the other—right, left, right, left—looking straight ahead and not saying a word. I felt bad for not acknowledging all the encouragement and kind remarks, but I knew that silent focus was the only way I was going to make it to the finish line.

Finally, I could see the finish line. The finish line! The finish line! A huge arch hung over the line. I loved that arch and everything it represented. *Just run to the arch. Run to the arch. The arch! Keep going! I am making it. I am going to make it!*

I ran under the arch and collapsed into my husband's arms. There was no one else around. The announcer was gone. The awards ceremony was already over. The crowds had all gone home. The race organizers were cleaning up. All the metal sawhorses had been removed from the transition area except the one on which my bike was hanging. They had even posted the "final" results. The only people around were my husband, the timer, and one kind man who clapped for me as I ran across the finish line.

But I didn't care. I had finished. I conquered the course. I was a triathlete. The deep joy of accomplishment was indescribable. I had overcome my fears and succeeded in something I had never thought I could do. It was the best feeling in the world.

When the results came out, I saw that it had taken me over two hours to complete the course. In comparison, the fastest woman finished in less than an hour, and the average woman finished in about an hour and a half. My time was super slow, but I didn't care. I had finished. In photos we took after the race, I am holding up my finisher's medal and one finger in victory. In my mind, I was number one.

As soon as I got home, I signed up for another triathlon. This time, I had two goals: to cross the finish line and to do so in less time than my first triathlon. In that race, I didn't brush my hair or eat a sandwich in transition. When the results were posted, I saw I had improved my time by ten minutes. That felt great. And then I noticed something else. I was second in my age group. During the awards ceremony, I grinned ear to ear when they called my name and I walked in front of everyone to receive my award.

I signed up for three more triathlons that summer and finished first in my age group in each. At first, I was elated. Then I realized that in these small local races, I was often the only one in my age group. It was pretty easy to be first when you're the only one. Sometimes I crossed the finish line last out of all the people who raced, but since I was the only one in my age group, I received a first-place medal. The win didn't feel like much of an accomplishment, since I hadn't really beaten anyone.

But then I realized that winning takes two things. First, you must cross the start line. Second, you must cross the finish line. As I stepped on the podium, I told myself that my medal represented the courage I had to cross the start line and the tenacity I demonstrated by making it to the finish line. At the same time, I was curious about my ability and wished I could race against other women my age to give some perspective to my performance. Little did I know that I would have that opportunity in my second triathlon season.

TRIATHLON SEASON 2

DISCOVERING ME

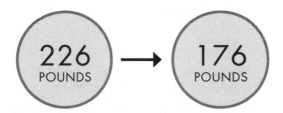

226 POUNDS → 176 POUNDS

Chapter 5

BECOMING COACHABLE

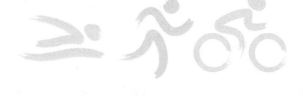

After the last race of my first season, I started thinking about the future. I knew I wanted to continue racing in triathlons, and I hoped to keep achieving personal bests, but I didn't know how to get faster. I thought about a coach but didn't think coaches were for people like me, an obese grandma. I wondered if I could get a triathlon coach to just sit down with me one time to give me some pointers.

An online search for "triathlon coach" brought up a group called USA Triathlon, the governing body for triathlon in the United States. Their website included a place where I could search for a certified coach in my area. My search produced one coach: Brant Bahler.

By searching on his name, I found the website for his company, Dream Big Triathlon Coaching. Coach Brant's accomplishments impressed me. His bio said he was a top-tier athlete who had played sports at a Division I college and was in the top three overall (not just in his age group) at many triathlons. It further described him as an Ironman and coach of people training for Ironman triathlons. I became intimidated. I didn't think a coach at his level would be interested in talking to me, a non-athlete who could barely run three miles. But I also noted that Coach Brant had received several mental-attitude awards in high school. As a former teacher, I knew mental-attitude awards usually go to students who are kind, positive, and enjoy helping others. I hoped Coach Brant fit that stereotype and might agree to talk with me.

I felt nervous about meeting face-to-face with someone I had found online but hadn't been introduced to, so I did a little more homework. The website said Coach Brant worked at our local YMCA and received their Employee of the Year award. I called the YMCA, and thankfully, they verified that Coach Brant is a good guy.

Finally, I reached out to Coach Brant. I sent an email to introduce myself and ask if he would be willing to talk with me. I described myself honestly in the email, and I wondered what Coach Brant would think when he read about my old age, big size, and lack of fitness. I thought he might simply click the trash icon, but within minutes, I had a response. Coach Brant said he'd love to talk and suggested that we meet. We set a time and place, and I started writing down all my questions.

On the day of our meeting, I became intimidated once again. I didn't feel worthy of Coach Brant's attention. I assumed that once he saw my obese body in person, he'd make an excuse and flee. Even worse, I feared he'd laugh at my dreams. As I drove to meet Coach Brant, I repeated the words that helped when I was scared: *Go away, fear. Go away, pride.*

Coach Brant met me at the door. I had seen photos of him online, but in person, his youthful appearance and obvious fitness made me feel even more intimidated. After saying hello, he suggested we go up to his office. I immediately zoned in on the word *up* and wondered if that meant stairs. Yes, it did. As I followed Coach Brant up the stairs, my heart started racing and my breathing became out of control. By the top step, I was gasping for air and knew I wouldn't be able to talk. When we sat down, I pointed to a photo on his desk and managed to say, "Your kids?" as my heart still hammered in my chest from the climb. While Coach Brant talked about his daughter and two sons, I forced myself to breath slowly and silently begged my heartrate to slow down. I hoped Coach Brant hadn't noticed my lack of fitness, but I suspected he had and now wondered why he had ever agreed to meet with an obese woman who couldn't even climb one flight of stairs.

To my relief, Coach Brant seemed nice and made talking easy. He didn't laugh or get up to flee. In fact, he behaved as if he wanted to talk to me. He patiently answered all my questions and explained the different ways that he could help me with triathlon. I'm not sure how it happened, but before I left, I had agreed to a coaching package. I now had a coach.

As soon as I got home, I sent Coach Brant another email outlining all the reasons that he might want to reconsider coaching me. I was old. I weighed a lot. I lacked fitness. I wanted to give him an opportunity to back out in case he'd had second thoughts. He wrote back, "I was born to coach." Somehow, those words made everything OK.

Our arrangement worked well. Each Sunday we exchanged emails: I sent Coach Brant a short summary of how the workouts had gone during the previous week, and then he sent me an email explaining what I had done well and where I needed to improve. This served as an accountability system similar to the one I'd had at Meltdown Bootcamp.

Coach Brant's emails also included my workouts for the coming week. The workouts he assigned were customized to my schedule, my goals, and my fitness level. On Sundays, I waited with eager anticipation for his email to arrive in my in-box. I wondered what new adventures I'd find in my workouts for the coming week.

Each day's workout included the sport I should do, the distance to cover, and how fast to go. Some days, Coach Brant would have me do a long distance at a slow pace. Other days, he'd tell me repeat a short distance multiple times at a fast pace with rests in between. Coach Brant also included a weekly motivational statement from great athletes and philosophers, like Aristotle's "Quality is not an act, it is a habit." On his website, he'd often add his own thoughts to the quotes. In this case, he wrote, "If you want to reach your big dreams, it takes relentless pursuit, a habit of the highest quality of commitment you can give. It takes not just short term periods of production, but a lifestyle of giving your best." The arrival of Coach Brant's weekly email filled me with excitement. I couldn't wait to see what he had planned for the week and be inspired by his quotes.

After the first few weeks of working together, I suddenly stopped sending emails. Pressures at work were taking a toll on me. I started backing away from everything else, including triathlon. I didn't realize how much I had disappeared until I received an email from Coach Brant that asked, "Are You OK?" in the subject line. In the body of the email, Coach Brant wrote, "Haven't heard from you. Is everything OK? I want to help, but I can't if I don't know what's going on."

I had known Coach Brant for only a few weeks. How did he know that something was wrong? I was impressed that rather than responding with irritation at my lack of responsibility, his words reflected kindness and compassion. I explained things were crazy at work and said, "I'm still motivated. Please don't give up on me." He responded, "I won't ever give up." At the time, I didn't know how true that statement would prove to be.

When things settled down at work in the late fall, I sent Coach Brant an email to let him know I was ready to start training again. I had been thinking about how much I struggled in the run and wondered if participating in a longer run event in the spring would build my confidence and make the triathlon's three miles seem easy. Later, after one of my workouts with Coach Brant, I asked what he thought about me running in the OneAmerica 500 Festival Mini-Marathon, the half-marathon race associated with the Indianapolis 500 car race in May. Coach Brant would have six months to train me for the 13.1-mile race. He hesitated. I could sense the wheels churning in his brain as he wondered about preparing an obese person who could barely run three miles for a half marathon. Finally, he said yes. He thought it was doable. He wanted to go for it. We started training for the half marathon.

• • •

At that time, Coach Brant was twenty-seven years old, younger than my sons. I felt motherly toward him like I do toward my sons and my sons' friends. But in reality, Coach Brant wasn't like a son at all. As my coach, he had authority over me. He told me what to do and expected me to do it—and scolded me from time to time when I didn't follow his instructions. I wasn't used to having someone so young giving me instructions, and I don't think Coach Brant was used to that either. Once he thanked me for taking directions from someone so young. But we both knew that if I was going to improve in triathlon, I needed to follow his lead. I was impressed that Coach Brant had the confidence he needed to coach someone twice his age.

I never minded when Coach Brant scolded me. I knew that his scolding came from a place of caring and he always scolded me gently. I think he understood that it wouldn't take much to get me to pay attention. I suspect he also realized that if he scolded too harshly, I would fall apart. When I failed to execute one of his workouts properly, he'd write "Sue!!!!" in his weekly feedback. When I saw four explanation points, I knew I'd messed up, and would read the next sentence carefully to see what I had done wrong. I found myself wanting to please Coach Brant and working for his praise.

Usually, the four exclamation points were a result of me doing more than the workout stated. As a student and employee, I had always tried to do a little bit more than my teachers and bosses asked of me. In those situations, going the extra mile had been appreciated. I did the same thing in training. If Coach Brant asked me to run two miles, I'd run three. I expected to receive praise for the extra mile, but would see "Sue!!!!" instead with a reminder to follow the workout as planned. It took me a while to understand that more is not better in athletic training.

Other times, I added distance or intensity to the workout because early in our coach-athlete relationship, I didn't trust that Coach Brant knew what he was doing. I read that runners preparing for half marathons should increase their longest run distance for the week by 10 percent each week. We weren't doing that so I started running extra miles. Once again, I saw "Sue!!!!" in Coach Brant's feedback, with strict instructions to not run farther than he said. When I told him that I was nervous because my longest runs weren't 10 percent longer each week and feared I wouldn't be ready for the half marathon, he patiently explained that he was splitting the distance into multiple short runs throughout the week. The sum of all the shorter distances would increase each week and I'd be prepared to run the 13.1 miles on race day without becoming injured. I hoped he was right, but I had my doubts.

Sometimes, Coach Brant scolded me in person and I found it so hard not to laugh. There's just something humorous about a twenty-seven-year-old scolding a grandma. One time during a run test, Coach Brant told me to do laps on a track until he told me to stop. With each lap, I was supposed to increase my speed just a little. I followed his instructions, but when Coach Brant told me to stop, I kept going and yelled back, "I have another gear in me!" When I stopped after finishing the extra lap, Coach Brant was not happy.

We stood face-to-face as he explained that I needed to be coachable. I needed to follow his instructions. I felt like a three-year-old who had been caught misbehaving and lowered my eyes as he talked. Then I started feeling tickled. The mental image of this serious young man scolding me, an old lady, made me want to laugh. I knew laughing was an inappropriate response for the situation, and I pressed my lips together. But I could not control the corners of my mouth, and they turned upward as I tried hard not to laugh. When I looked at Coach Brant, I could see the corners of his mouth turning up, too. He walked away so I wouldn't see him smile. We were both tickled.

I never faulted Coach Brant for being firm with me, because I knew it came from a kind place. He wanted me to reach my goals because he cared about me. He was simply telling me what I needed to hear. I wanted that in a coach.

• • •

As we continued to prepare for the half marathon in May, I began striving to do every workout exactly as written, even on holidays. On New Year's Eve, I ran up a steep hill and then walked down, over and over, while striving to keep my heart rate below a certain level during the climbs. I wore a heart rate monitor and set an alarm on my sports watch so it would give a series of shrill beeps if I pushed too hard and caused my heart rate to go too high. The workout went well with no beeps, and I jogged home to send Coach Brant my feedback.

As I sat writing, my sports watch suddenly started alarming. I had forgotten to turn it off. I looked at the heart rate, and it was sky-high—about twice what it should have been. I figured my sports watch had malfunctioned and took my heart rate manually. Holding my wrist, I counted the beats for ten seconds and then multiplied by six. The result was the same number as my sports watch displayed. Evidently, my heart was beating at twice its normal rate.

I explained the situation to my husband, and he thought I might be having a heart attack, but I felt no pain. To be safe, we decided to go to the walk-in clinic, so they could check me out. I left my sports watch on to continuing monitor my heart rate and hoped it would go back to normal before we arrived at the clinic. That was not the case.

Everyone in the clinic looked up as I walked in the door with my sports watch screaming BEEP! BEEP! BEEP! After I explained my situation to the receptionist, she seemed a little panicked and rushed me to an examination room. The next thing I knew, I was on a table with electrodes all over my body. I later learned that people with heart issues usually go directly to the emergency room, so prompt-med clinics don't have a lot of experience with heart emergencies. After confirming my unusually high heart rate and determining that I was not in immediate danger of dying, they told my husband to drive me to our hospital's emergency room.

The hospital receptionist immediately sent me to an examination room, and once again, I lay in a bed with electrodes all over my body. However, no doctors were available. I had to wait for hours, and during that time, my heart returned to normal without any interventions. For the first time ever, I was glad to wait a long time to see a doctor. When the doctor finally arrived, she said I might have been dehydrated and sent me home with instructions to follow up with my doctor.

I sent a text to Coach Brant to explain what had happened. He wrote back immediately, "Tell me what you need, and I will do it." There was something about the wording of his text that touched me deeply. It was so much more than "Let me know if you need anything." Coach Brant commanded me, "Tell me what you need," and then promised, "and I will do it." At that moment, I understood the degree to which Coach Brant cared about me as a person. It wasn't just about triathlon.

A few days later, I saw my internist, the same one who earlier had told me not to run, and he told me to see a cardiologist. After several tests, including a stress test, my cardiologist told me I had experienced an atrial flutter (not the more serious atrial fibrillation), and it was probably just a freak thing. By chance, my cardiologist was also a distance runner. I suspect it gave him great pleasure to give me permission to start running again. My heart never fluttered again (except when my husband was around, of course).

Coach Brant and I resumed working together. He told me what to do during training, how much to sleep, and what to wear. One day after a track workout, he said in all seriousness, "You need a tighter bra." Evidently, I was bouncing as I ran, and he felt the bouncing might slow me down. I tried not to laugh at the image of a young coach talking to a grandma about her bouncing boobs, but this time I couldn't contain myself. I laughed and laughed.

A week before the race, I was a wreck. I had been training hard for months, and it was all coming down to one day—race day. I didn't know it then, but I was displaying typical pre-race jitters. Every time

I sneezed, I thought I had pneumonia. When I stubbed my toe, I was sure I had broken a bone in my foot. And worst of all, I started being cranky at home. For a few days, my poor husband had to put up with a wife who had no patience as I struggled with my fears about being able to finish the 13.1 miles.

Coach Brant gave me a race plan that instructed me to alternate five minutes of running with one minute of walking throughout the race. He also told me to drink water constantly and eat a gel (a little packet of sweet goop with the consistency of jam and one hundred calories) every thirty minutes.

The day before the race, Coach Brant sent me a kind note that filled me with calmness. On race morning, I wrote parts of his note on a little piece of paper: "Relax. Follow the Plan. Smile." I added the names of three people I wanted to remember for inspiration during the race. I had one granddaughter at the time and one on the way, so two of the names were Harper and Emma Kate. I hoped to set an example for them and other grandchildren that I might have in the future.

The other name was Tom Morris, a young strength coach at Indiana University. While mountain biking, he had experienced a horrendous crash that left him paraplegic. I had read about Tom's journey online. After the crash, he lay on the forest floor, unable to move, until someone found him. Over difficult months, he fought his way to self-sufficiency in a wheelchair and returned to his job at the university. I felt deeply moved by his courage, mental strength, and ability to withstand pain. When my training runs became difficult, I thought of him and kept going. Now I would think of him during my race.

I folded the piece of paper into a little square and put it in my pocket to carry with me while I ran the 13.1 miles. If I started to struggle during the race, I planned to pull out that piece of paper and draw inspiration from the names it contained.

But luckily, I didn't need it. I followed Coach Brant's race plan and felt great for the entire run. My excitement overflowed when I reached the ten-mile marker. *I am going to make it! Oh, my gosh! I am going to make it!* I couldn't believe nothing hurt, and I started to appreciate my training and my coach.

I thought the last three miles would be the worst, but being so close to the finish line created energy and kept me going. I noticed a distinct change in the people around me. At the start of the race, everyone had been running, chatting, and laughing. Now everyone walked, and no one was saying a word. People were dog tired—but I felt great.

With the finish line only three miles away, I found myself running faster. I tried not to overdo it, but when I looked at my sports watch, I saw that my pace was two minutes per mile faster than my planned pace. I forced myself to slow down but still ran slightly over my planned pace. My form felt good. My body felt good. Everything felt great.

When I turned the corner onto New York Street for Victory Mile, everyone started getting excited. We had been running for three hours, and there was just one mile left. Spectators on both sides of the street were waving flags and yelling, "One more mile!" The runners were yelling, "One more mile!" The volunteers were yelling, "One more mile!" I was yelling, "One more mile!"

New York Street had two hills, and I had preplanned to walk up both of them. I wanted so badly to run, but I forced myself to walk. There was no use sending my heart rate soaring at this point. But as soon as things leveled out, I ran with gusto—feet planted below my hips, head up, arms back. I felt *so* good.

At the time, I didn't know that runners were not allowed to carry cell phones, and I had taken mine with me in case something went wrong and I needed to call my husband. I pulled out my cell phone and called my husband. He immediately asked in panic, "What's wrong?!"

"Nothing," I quickly replied in a voice filled with excitement. "I am coming down the home stretch. Woohoo! I'm going to make it! See you in a few minutes!" The woman next to me overheard my end of the conversation and started laughing. "Isn't this fun?" I asked excitedly. She agreed, and we ran down the road with huge smiles on our faces.

Finally, I ran in front of stands filled with cheering spectators at the finish line. Black and white checkered flags lined the road, and the roar of race cars filled the air as the public-address system blasted soundtracks from past Indy 500 finishes. Vroom! Vroom! All the walkers started running toward the finish banner that hung over the road. We were all going to make it!

In my 5K races, I had always sprinted to the finish line. But this time, I wanted to savor the moment. Keeping a steady pace, I ran down the finish chute, shouting, "Woohoo!" over and over. With my hands in the air, I stepped across the finish line and yelled in excitement, "I did it!" Then I choked up a bit. I had run a half marathon.

I couldn't wait to tell Coach Brant, so I sent him a text before the finisher's medal had even been placed around my neck. My first text simply said, "Finished!!!!" Then I wrote, "We did it!!!! Followed the plan the whole way. Feel great! You are the BEST coach!"

Coach Brant texted back, "I am the proudest coach in town!" I was filled with sheer joy. I had made my coach proud. Nothing could have made me happier at that moment. I wanted him to be proud—not of me, but of his accomplishment. He took an obese, sixty-year-old woman and turned her into a half-marathoner. What an amazing accomplishment for him. We had done it together—his plan, my execution. We were a team.

I walked between two rows of booths, where water and recovery foods were being distributed to the tired runners. As I walked, I called my son Andy and babbled in happiness as I held a half-eaten banana in one hand and my phone in the other. I thanked him for encouraging me to enter that first 5K, and then I started to cry. I had come so far and felt so many emotions—joy, satisfaction, and gratitude for all who helped me along the way.

That deep satisfaction was becoming a familiar feeling at finish lines. It didn't matter where I placed. The satisfaction came from knowing I had done my best. I had trained every day for months for the half marathon and, more importantly, had overcome my fears. *I nailed the race.*

That evening, Coach Brant posted a photo of me wearing my finisher's medal on his Facebook page, along with these words: "I can't say enough about this special lady. This race finish was a huge step in a journey in her quest for a healthier life. To date, Sue has lost over 140 lbs. She has worked so hard to get where she is, and we aren't done yet! She will tell you I was a big part of her success, but a coach is nothing without an athlete that is willing to listen, learn, and then follow it up with dedication and hard work. One very proud coach today!" I went to bed with a happy heart.

My performance in the OneAmerica 500 Festival Mini-Marathon brought my trust in Coach Brant to a new level. I had crossed the half-marathon finish line with a smile on my face, uninjured, and with enough energy to run another thirteen miles. I now believed in Coach Brant's training and knew he would always have me ready for my races when I stood on the start line. In the summer months that followed the race, that trust would become key as I began competing in large triathlons and discovered an athlete hiding inside.

Chapter 6

FACING FEAR, FINDING COURAGE

With May's half marathon behind me, I refocused my training on triathlon, with the goal of increasing my fitness and improving technique in swim, bike, and run. Hopefully, I would be faster in the coming months as I raced in my second triathlon season. I completed daily workouts assigned by Coach Brant, although I missed a few when life got in the way. My training paid off, and I set personal records in the first few races I entered for the season. The improvement excited me, and after each race, I posted on Facebook, "Woohoo! Another PR!"

While I enjoyed racing against myself, I continued to wonder how I compared with other women my age. I wanted to understand my skill level better, and to do that, I needed a perspective I didn't get when I was the only one in my age group during a race. I also found it difficult to see improvement. Sure, my times were getting faster. But in triathlon, where the course and weather change each week, differences in finish times are not reliable indicators of improvement. Sometimes you're faster because the weather is cooler or the run course has fewer climbs.

I finally decided to compare myself with all women who participated in the race, not just those in my age group. That didn't help me understand how my performance compared with others my age, but if I improved, I would be able to see myself move up in rank within the large group of all women. The first time I calculated my rank, I was at the ninety-ninth percentile. In other words, I was dead last. But as my workouts made me stronger and fitter, and as I learned more about triathlon technique, my rank among all women started to improve. Slowly, I moved from ninety-ninth to ninetieth percentile, then eightieth. I felt thrilled when I hit the seventy-fifth percentile; I was no longer in the bottom quarter. As my rank climbed, I knew Coach Brant and I were on the right track, but I still didn't know how I compared with other women my age.

My love of triathlon was growing. I started following the world's fastest triathletes who traveled around the world to compete in a collection of races called the World Triathlon Series sponsored by the International Triathlon Union (ITU), the organization that coordinates triathlon on an international basis. At each of the races, the top competitors received points based on how they placed, and at the end of the year, the athlete with the most points was crowned world champion. My favorite triathlete was Gwen Jorgensen, who in 2016 became the first American to win the Olympic gold medal in triathlon. I loved Gwen's focus on the process of improvement and her humble yet hungry attitude. Although Gwen was half my age, we had started doing triathlons at about the same time. In just a few years, she went from triathlon newbie to Olympic championship. She inspired me to the moon and back.

ITU announced that one of the races in the series would be held in Chicago. The World Triathlon Chicago race would be just four hours from my home, and I decided to attend so I could watch Gwen and all the other top triathletes who were hoping for positions on their country's Olympic triathlon team. Later, I learned that in addition to the race for the elite triathletes, an open race would be held for age-groupers like me. My wheels started rolling. I couldn't stop thinking about the possibility of racing in an international event with thousands of triathletes from around the world. The idea of racing on the same course as Gwen Jorgensen (though on a different day) felt crazy-exciting.

I wrote to Coach Brant, "What do you think about me racing in the open race at the World Triathlon Series when it comes to Chicago? I know I will come in last (or second-to-last based on last year's times). I don't care about being last. However, I don't want to put people out. Do you think people will be inconvenienced by my slow times? Will my slowness endanger others? Will I be in people's way? Will people swim over me? Bike over me? Is this a good idea?"

Later, Coach Brant and I talked face-to-face, and I asked my questions again. He hesitated. We only had two months to prepare, and he worried that the sheer size of the event would be incredibly overwhelming for a virtual beginner. Finally, he gave me the go-ahead. As soon as I got the green light, I registered for the race before I could chicken out. So for the next two months, Coach Brant wrote workouts to prepare me for my first large race.

A few days before leaving for Chicago, I received an email from ITU, warning that the water temperature in Lake Michigan, where we would be swimming, was a frigid fifty-five degrees Fahrenheit. The email strongly suggested that race participants wear wet suits during the swim to stay warm. I didn't own a wet suit, but I knew what they looked like. They were black and skintight, covered every inch of your body, and appeared to be made out of old car tires. Their purpose was to keep you warm.

I called some triathlon shops in Indianapolis, but no one had my plus-size in stock. With the race just a few days away, I called Blue Seventy, one of the better-known wet-suit manufacturers. Thankfully, they agreed to send me wet suits in three different sizes, so I could try them on. When they arrived, I tried on the smallest wet suit first. My husband helped me pull the black, rubbery fabric over my legs and arms. But once I had it on, it felt so tight that I couldn't move, and we laughed as I walked around the living room like a toy soldier. The middle-size wet suit seemed to fit the best, but I wasn't sure. I called Coach Brant, and he suggested that we meet at the YMCA pool so he could check it out.

In the locker room, I put on the wet suit over my bathing suit. But I couldn't reach the long zipper in the back. With no one around to help, I walked out to the pool deck with the back unzipped. When Coach Brant saw me, he pinched the fabric on my arms and told me he thought it fit well but that I didn't have it pulled up enough to allow my shoulders to move freely. He instructed me to turn away from him, and then with two hands, he grabbed the open zipper and pulled up hard. The motion jerked my feet off the ground and gave me a huge wedgie, but the suit ended up where it needed to be, and I could freely move my shoulders and arms. I've since learned that there's an art to putting on a tight-fitting wet suit, and the last step is always asking my husband to give me a wedgie.

Once I had the wet suit on properly, Coach Brant told me to jump into the deep end of the pool. Nervously, I looked at the water. I knew a lot of people had trouble swimming in a wet suit. The tightness of the fabric makes them feel as if they can't breathe, and many, even competent swimmers, have panic attacks in the water. I wasn't sure how I would react in the water with the wet suit squeezing me on all sides.

I jumped in and immediately came flying to the surface. The foamy wet-suit material seemed like a full-length life preserver. Without even kicking, I floated vertically, with my head and shoulders above the water. My body just bobbed up and down, like a fishing bobber. It was such a funny feeling that I burst out laughing.

I swam a few lengths and was amazed that my legs stayed at the top of the water without much kicking. Swimming in a wet suit was fun. It would also be fast, since my legs would drag less in the water. And while I sensed pressure all around, I never felt that I couldn't breathe. I loved my wet suit.

Having resolved the issue of the wet suit, I had to figure out what to take to the race. Chicago was four hours away—too far to run home if I forgot something. I wrote down everything I'd need and came up with long list. I checked off each item as I put it in one of several suitcases. When possible, I also packed backups in case something essential, like swim goggles, broke or got lost. I also packed the food I would eat the night before, the morning of, and during the race.

I studied the race plan Coach Brant gave me, along with the race maps the race director provided. The swim would start near Buckingham Fountain. We'd swim 0.5 miles along the Lake Michigan shoreline and get out of the water by the Shedd Aquarium. Then we'd run a half mile to transition, where we'd pick up our bike and ride 12.4 miles on closed roads in downtown Chicago. Once back to transition, we'd rack our bike and then run 3.1 miles through Chicago, winding up at Buckingham Fountain.

My husband and I planned to arrive in Chicago a few days before the race, and I looked online for a Lake Michigan beach near the race start where I could practice swimming. I had never raced 0.5 miles in the swim before. In my previous races, the race directors had all shortened the swim to make their races more beginner friendly. I had never raced in a large body of water where there could be significant waves. I had never raced in a wet suit. And if that wasn't enough, this race had a mass start. Instead of entering the water one at a time, the 150 women in my wave would all tread water together. Then a horn would blast, and we'd all take off with elbows flying, feet kicking, and water churning. Luckily, I'm comfortable in the water, but having never seen or experienced this type of race start before, I felt scared. I found a nearby beach for practice, but it was closed due to water quality. Now I had another concern to add to my growing list: water pollution.

When my husband and I arrived in Chicago, we drove the bike and run courses twice. On the first trip, I read the map and told Brian where to turn as we followed the course. On the second trip, we put the map away, and I told him where to turn from memory.

The bike course terrified me. In the United States, bike courses usually involve riding six miles away from transition and then riding six miles back. However, the international races sponsored by ITU usually have a looped course, where riders ride around a short loop multiple times. This makes the race more interesting for spectators, who see the bikes go by several times. However, it makes the course more dangerous, since hundreds of bikes are all bunched up on less road surface. But those weren't the only things that concerned me about the bike course. To my horror, I discovered that a third of the bike course would be underground.

About halfway through each loop, the course went down a ramp to Lower Wacker Drive, an underground highway beneath the city of Chicago. I wondered how my eyes would adjust from the bright sunlight to the darkness of the tunnel, and I imagined racing blindly while my eyes adjusted. Once underground, we would race past cement pillars and walls that were just a few feet away. If someone went down in that section of the course, they would smack into cement. For the millionth time, I thought about backing out. But then I said to myself, *OK. If you die, you die. You are doing this race.*

After reviewing the route, Brian and I checked into our hotel, and I sent Coach Brant an email with a few questions about the race but didn't hear back from him. The next morning, we walked to Grant Park, where I would pick up my registration packet. Triathlon vendors had set up tents in the park and were selling all sorts of triathlon gear: clothing, nutrition products, technology. In the registration tent, volunteers sat behind boxes at a long table. Each box contained registration packets, and long lines of triathletes stretched from each box. I found the box that included the *R*s and got in line.

While I waited, an ITU official walked by, and I stopped him to ask a question: "I'm a beginner and was wondering—" He interrupted me, "If you're a beginner, you probably shouldn't be here." My struggling confidence sank to a new low. Tears ran down my cheeks. Inside my head, my rational mind and my irrational mind started an argument:

"That official shouldn't have said that. He is a jerk."

"Yeah, but he's right. You are in way over your head. Back out now."

"But you've come all this way. You are here."

"Yeah, but do you really want to ride underground on your bike next to cement walls?"

"The odds of getting hurt are slim. Remember what your brother said: 'Race directors don't plan dangerous races. They want everyone to be safe. They don't want to be sued.' You're staying. End of discussion."

Thankfully, my rational mind won that conversation. Although scared to the bone, I remained in line and accepted my race packet from the volunteer. When we got back to the hotel, I checked to see if there was a message from Coach Brant, hoping he'd help me calm down, but no reply had arrived.

That afternoon, we went to see the elite women race. I couldn't wait to see Gwen Jorgensen on the race course. We left early to get a good position at the swim start. On the walk to the start, I glanced to my right and was shocked to see Gwen Jorgensen walking beside me. I wanted to say, "Gwen Jorgensen! You are my hero!" Instead, I just watched as she talked quietly with a man who I assumed was her coach. The conversation was very calm and serious. He seemed to be sharing last-minute reminders about the race. The two of them seemed oblivious to everything going on around them. A few people shouted, "Go, Gwen!" as we walked the two blocks to the swim start, but she didn't respond. She was in race mode.

I was amazed by how close we could get to the elite athletes. At the swim start, I stood about ten feet away from Gwen and took close-up photos with my phone. During her run, I could stand right at the edge of the course. At one point, I leaned over the railing to take a photo of Gwen as she approached. As I started to take the photo, I found that I had misjudged how fast she was running, and we almost collided. I ended up with a photo of Gwen's stomach with

"JORGENSEN USA" written across it. I refrained from leaning over the railing after that. Gwen won her race. Go, USA!

My race was the next day. That night, I ate the spaghetti we brought from home and checked my email. Still no response from Coach Brant. Discouraged by my fears and the official's remarks, I figured Coach Brant was too busy with his "real" athletes, seasoned triathletes who were participating in an Ironman the next day, to have time for me, a beginner who was in over her head. At that point, I didn't know Coach Brant well enough to understand that all of his athletes get his attention, not just those doing Ironman races.

As I continued thinking about my race the next day, I started to have a major meltdown. "I can't do this," I sobbed. "What was I thinking?" I entered that dark place of self-doubt and fear. My sweet husband tried to help, but his advice was "If this scares you, maybe you shouldn't do it." I think he felt scared, too. I desperately wanted to ask Coach Brant questions, and once again, I thought about backing out. I felt seriously in over my head. I wasn't a real athlete. I was an imposter—just an old lady who thought she could do more than she could. At this point, my irrational mind was winning the debate. I didn't know what to do.

Then my phone buzzed. It was a text from Coach Brant. Hallelujah! He apologized for not getting back to me sooner. Somehow, he had missed my emails. He asked how things were going.

I found myself torn between wanting to project an "I have it all together" image and wanting to burst into tears and admit that I was a mess. Luckily, we were texting, so I could do both. As tears streamed down my face, I typed questions that I hoped would give the impression I was in control. But when I started telling him about the ITU official who told me I didn't belong at the race because I was a beginner, Coach Brant saw through me. He started telling me all the reasons that I *should* be at that race. I was strong. I was prepared. I was ready. I needed to follow the plan that he had laid out, and I would be fine. He also answered the technical questions I had about the course. Slowly, I started to believe in myself again. I remembered who I was and what I was capable of doing. I told pride and fear to go away. I might come in dead last, but I belonged there.

The next morning, I arrived at the swim start at 10:00 to get ready for my 12:10 wave. The heat was brutal. ITU race officials assess the heat injury risk by monitoring the heat, humidity, and wind. They post different-colored flags and make announcements to alert race participants about the risk level. Right before my wave, the risk was upgraded from green to yellow, and we were told to hydrate well during the race. With a temperature of 85 degrees Fahrenheit and 84 percent humidity, the air felt like a sauna.

When they called my wave, I entered a corral with all the women who were around my age. After a short wait, we were told to jump into the fifty-five-degree water. The freezing water stung my bare feet, hands, and face, but it felt good to be out of the heat. I positioned myself toward the back and then treaded water with the other women waiting for the start horn to blast. I could not contain my excitement. I had conquered my fears and was about to start. I was on top of the world. I yelled, "Woohoo!" Then the woman next to me yelled, "Woohoo!" and suddenly everyone was yelling, "Woohoo!" I will never forget that moment.

The horn blasted, and I began swimming along the shoreline of Lake Michigan. On my first breath, I inhaled water and was grateful that I knew what to do. I stayed calm, held my breath until the choking spasm subsided, and then took another breath. Other than that, it was an uneventful swim, and I enjoyed watching the people on the shore as I turned my head for air. At the end of the swim, we were supposed to climb up a steep ramp to get out of the water. But before I even stopped swimming, a volunteer grabbed me by the armpits and literally threw me up the ramp.

The bike was a blast. I sped along Columbus Drive and noted that I passed some strong-looking young men who were wearing pointy aero helmets. That I was passing them made no sense to me, but I didn't complain.

As I feared, the transition from daylight to darkness when we rode underground caused temporary blindness, but it lasted only a few seconds. Luckily, no one made unexpected moves while our eyes adjusted. However, there were crashes underground. I passed two ambulances whose EMTs were helping riders who had crashed into the cement pillars. That scared me, but I had to stay focused on my own race so while hoping they were OK, I put them out of my mind. After the race, I tried to find out if they were OK, but no one knew. I assumed they weren't hurt too badly, since no one had information about injuries.

While I loved the bike portion of the race, the run was another story. It was scorching hot. I had never raced in heat before, and I didn't know how heat impacts one's performance. My slow pace puzzled me. I figured I wasn't putting in enough effort, so I ran harder, but that didn't make any difference. I was still slow. I thought maybe I needed calories, so I started eating the gels I was carrying with me. That didn't help either. To make matters worse, part of the run course was paved with white granite blocks. The heat radiating up from the granite felt even hotter than the heat blaring down from the sun.

ITU had placed big fans periodically along the run course. The fans sprayed a cool mist on the runners, but every time I approached one, a group of racers stood directly in front of it as they tried to cool off, so I just ran by. I kept thinking I would speed up, but every time I tried, it was a no go. The heat won. I was cooked, but thankfully, I crossed the finish line.

A short while later, Coach Brant called. He said the race results were already posted online, and he sounded excited. He told me there were sixteen women in the sixty-to-sixty-four age group. For the first time, I would be able to compare myself with other women my age. I was tenth! Almost in the top half! I finished fourth in the swim and seventh in the bike. I finally knew how I compared with other women my age, and I felt ecstatic to be so close to the middle of the pack.

Later that evening, I thought about all the fears I had conquered in Chicago. My fears all seemed to start with one of two phrases: "what if" or "yeah, but": *What if I inconvenience the volunteers? What if I can't breathe in my wet suit? What if I crash on my bike? Yeah, but I don't know how to do a mass start. Yeah, but I'm just a beginner.* I recognized that "what if" and "yeah, but" were red flags, alerting me of fears that could get in the way of my progress. I thought it might be a good idea to never say those words.

As I thought about my fears, I realized they each fit into one of three boxes. I labeled the first box Do Not Think about These Things. That box included irrational fears like being afraid of the unknown at the start of the bike segment. My logical mind knew the bike was going to be fine, but my fearful mind was sure I would crash into a cement pillar. My strategy for addressing irrational fears was to simply force myself to think about something else every time they popped into my head.

The second box was called Things I Can Control. It included fears I could identify and address ahead of time. For example, when I feared panic attacks caused by my wet suit, I went to the pool to get

used to swimming in a wet suit. To address my fear of hitting a pot-
hole on the bike course, I drove the course prior to the race to scout
for potholes. When I started worrying about my googles breaking at
the last minute, I brought a backup pair of goggles to the swim start.
These fears were manageable.

The last box was named Chaos. These fears were impossible to
predict and out of my control. In Chicago, a storm caused an unexpected change in the time and location for packet pickup. I had no
idea when or where to pick up the packet that included my race bib,
timing chip, and colored swim cap that corresponded to my swim
wave, and I panicked, using valuable energy. After that meltdown,
I decided to simply accept that chaos is part of racing. When the
unexpected happens, I tell myself to accept and adjust. First, I *accept*
that something unexpected occurred, and then I calmly *adjust* to the
situation. I may not be in control of the chaos, but I can be in control
of my reaction to chaos.

In Chicago, I learned a lot about racing that would help in future
races, and I developed confidence that I had the strength to face
scary situations and survive. But best of all, I learned where I stood
in triathlon among women my age. I started feeling a twinge of
excitement and a glimmer of hope, and I began to daydream in secret
once again. I wondered what would happen if I really committed to
triathlon. I was eager to race against women my age again and would
have that opportunity a month later at the USA Triathlon National
Championship.

Chapter 7

DISCOVERING THE
ATHLETE INSIDE

The USA Triathlon National Championship (commonly referred to as Nationals) was being held in Milwaukee a month after my race in Chicago. At that time, registration for the sprint-distance race at Nationals was open to anyone. I had signed up earlier in the summer so I'd have a second chance to race against women my age. Now I wondered if I could repeat the performance I'd had in Chicago and come close to the top half again. I wasn't so sure. At Nationals, the best triathletes in the country would be in attendance, racing for the national podium. Surely, I would be near the bottom. To help with speed, I purchased a new bike—a Cervélo S3.

Cervélo Cycles manufactures top-end bikes, and the S3 is one of their fastest road bikes. At the time, I didn't have the cycling experience to sense its responsiveness to my body's motions or appreciate the way its gears shifted so smoothly. That would come later. For now, I liked its red color with the word Cervélo in big white letters on the side of the frame, and I knew the lightness of the carbon frame would make me faster.

While the S3 was an amazing bike, it was not a triathlon bike. It didn't have the special aerodynamic handlebars (aerobars) that allow riders to rest their elbows on the bike to lower their upper body, resulting in less wind resistance. I decided not to add clip-in pedals that would allow me to attach my feet to the bike. Instead, I added platform pedals—similar to the pedals my sons had on their bikes when they were little boys. I also decided not to add wide-rimmed wheels to the bike. I knew clip-in pedals and wide-rim wheels would make me faster, but I feared they would also result in me taking a nasty fall.

I named my bike Red and told him he deserved a much better rider than me. I promised to take good care of him and explained that if he stuck with me, I would work hard to grow into the rider he deserved. My husband thought I was crazy to be talking to my bike, but almost all the triathletes do so. Your bike becomes your partner. Your muscles create power. The bike turns that power into forward motion. The more I rode Red, the more I fell in love him. I couldn't wait to ride Red at Nationals.

I was excited to have another chance to race against a large group of women in my age group and looked forward to observing the best women my age in the country. To be honest, I was kind of in awe of them. Some of them were like rock stars to me, especially Carol Hassell, who was ranked first in the nation.

After racing in Chicago, I wasn't as nervous. I now had experience with wetsuits and mass starts. But one thing about the Milwaukee race terrified me: the bike course would cross Hoan Bridge, a suspension bridge that spans two miles and rises 120 feet (twelve stories) over the Milwaukee River. Suspension bridges have always frightened me. I imagine myself going over the side and falling to my death. I am so afraid that I sometimes make my family drive miles out of our way on vacations so we don't have to cross one. When we do cross a suspension bridge, I close my eyes from start to finish, counting to one hundred over and over to keep my mind occupied.

To make matters worse, I learned that a portion of Hoan Bridge had given way a few years earlier after two of the three support beams failed, causing the lanes to buckle and sag by several feet. Experts worried that the whole bridge might collapse. Thinking about riding my bike over Hoan Bridge with only a small cement wall separating me and a 120-foot fall seemed like a nightmare.

I sent Coach Brant an email saying, "I am only going to say this one time, and then I am not going to bring it up again, because I don't want to breathe life into my fear. I am absolutely terrified of suspension bridges. I just want you to know." After that, I put Hoan Bridge into the mental box labeled Do Not Think about These Things. Every time I found myself thinking about Hoan Bridge, I forced my mind to think about something else. Coach Brant never said a thing about Hoan Bridge, but I noticed that hill repeats started appearing in my workouts, giving me confidence that I could at least climb the steep slope over Hoan Bridge.

Several days before the race, my husband and I drove to Milwaukee so I could check out the race venue and hopefully do a few workouts on the race course. As we drove, I composed a silly little song in my head and sang it to myself over and over: *I'm going to Milwaukee! I'm going to the race! To see the elite women set a record pace!* As soon as we arrived, we drove the bike course, so I could scout for potholes. That meant driving over Hoan Bridge. As we approached, I saw a road with a steep grade that seemed to go up forever, and my heart began racing. As the car started climbing up the ramp to the bridge, I remembered which fear box contained Hoan Bridge and started a new mantra, pausing after each word: *Do . . . not . . . think . . . about . . . these . . . things.* I hoped that mantra would also work on race day.

Two days before the race, we walked to packet pickup. I was surprised to receive a nice jacket with a USA Triathlon National Championship label on it. However, when I tried it on, it was way too big. I had registered months earlier and was now three sizes smaller. Luckily, I was able to exchange it. Then I looked at my timing chip and panicked. The number did not match my race number. I told myself, *This is race chaos. Accept and adjust.* Then I calmly found a race official. When I explained the situation, he abruptly and rather rudely told me, "Don't worry about it." Before I knew it, tears streamed down my cheeks. Instead of accepting and adjusting, I was fretting and fuming. I found another official and asked the same question, but before I could get out the last words, the tears came again, along with sobs. That's when I realized I had some significant fears about being in over my head at a national championship. Luckily, this official was as nice as could be. He took the time to answer my questions and explained that my timing chip was not a problem.

The afternoon before the race, my husband and I took my bike to transition, where I would leave it overnight. While racking my bike, I chatted with triathletes from across the country. Usually, the conversation opened with them saying something about my awesome bike. I realized that a Cervélo bike probably looked funny with platform pedals, so I'd explain that the bike was way beyond my skill level, but I was hoping to improve. People asked me where I was from and we launched new friendships as we shared our excitement for the race. Great fun.

That night after dinner, I had a major meltdown. As hard as I tried to keep Hoan Bridge out of my mind, it snuck out of the box and back into my consciousness. The anxieties began playing in my head: *I'm out of my league, not a national-level triathlete. I'm an impostor. I don't belong at this race.* I called Coach Brant, and once again he talked me back to reality. I was not going to fall off the bridge. I was strong. I was prepared. I should just follow the race plan, and everything would be fine.

Race morning went smoothly. I woke early, ate breakfast, and walked the few short blocks to the race with my husband. We put a blanket on the grass at Discovery World, close to the race start in Lake Michigan. I did my warm-up, received good-luck texts from my sons, and sent them a couple of photos. Then I put on my wet suit. Brian gave me a perfect wedgie, pulled the wet suit over my shoulders, and zipped up the back. I was ready to race.

As in Chicago, this race had a mass start, but instead of treading water, the 150 women in my wave put one hand on a dock that extended far into Lake Michigan. At the start of the swim, we spread out from left to right, but we quickly converged into one big mass of swimmers as we all swam toward the same point about 275 meters from the start: a narrow bridge that we would swim under.

The closer we got to the bridge, the more congested the water became with swimmers. People's hands were brushing my feet. Their hips were hitting my sides. Someone's fingernails clawed my hand. For a while, every time I breathed to my right, I was face-to-face with a woman who was breathing to her left. On one breath, she smiled at me. Amid all the pandemonium, that cracked me up. A little later, another woman hit me squarely in the face with her hand. It felt like she'd punched me with her fist. Ouch! The impact knocked off my goggles (and gave me a black eye). I did a few quick breaststroke kicks as I placed the goggles back on my face, and took off again.

Shortly after that, my life changed. I found myself swimming hip-to-hip with a woman as we raced for the opening of the little bridge. Our sides were rubbing against each other as we raced. And then my arm came down between her shoulder blades. I didn't know what to do. The kind thing would have been to pull back, say, "Oh, excuse me," and motion for her to go ahead. Instead, I continued my arm rotation as I raced. That motion literally shoved her underwater, and I swam over her as she disappeared below me. I reached the bridge first.

To my utter shock, I loved that moment of person-to-person physical competition. It exposed a primal, competitive instinct within me that I'd had no idea existed. That urge to dominate was opposite of the image I'd had of myself as a gentle, soft-spoken person. I didn't know it then, but I would spend considerable time after the race coming to terms with the competitive monster hiding inside of me.

The rest of the swim was fast and furious. Then I ran up the ramp that led us from the water to our bikes in the transition area, grabbed my bike, pushed it onto the bike course, and jumped on. Once I was on my bike, I forgot all about my fear of Hoan Bridge. In fact, when I started climbing Hoan Bridge, I didn't even realize I was on a bridge.

My hill repeats in training paid off, and I climbed the steep grade with ease. I was fearless on the downhill and pushed my bike to speeds approaching thirty-three miles per hour. I had practiced that, too. I wanted to make sure I didn't wimp out on the descents. On one descent, we were three abreast as I passed people who were passing other people. Still no fear. I loved speeding past everyone.

On the final descent, I knew there would be a big bump across the road where the city had placed a cover over an expansion grate to keep our bike wheels from falling through. From talking to Coach Brant about the bump, I knew I could hit the bump at full speed, provided I was square and steady on my bike. Right before contact, I made sure my front wheel was straight, stopped pedaling, and got ready to absorb the impact with my legs. Then, bang! The impact was jarring, but I stayed upright and flew past several other bikes that had slowed down. I wanted to yell, "Wheeeee!"

The run was beautiful. We ran in a park along Lake Michigan. The temperatures were warm but much cooler than they had been in Chicago, so my pace was where I expected it to be.

When the race was over and the results posted, I was pleased to see that I'd placed twenty-ninth in a field of forty-four women my age. Having two finishes near the middle of the pack at big races, I became even more curious about my triathlon future and asked the question again: What would happen if I really committed?

Then someone near the posted results told me that USA Triathlon invites the top eighteen women finishers in each age group at Nationals to be part of Team USA. Team USA members compete on behalf of the United States at the Age Group Triathlon World Championship (commonly referred to as Worlds). What an honor that would be! She added that people who place nineteenth through twenty-fifth become alternates for the team. If a Team USA member can't compete at Worlds, an alternate takes her place. Again, I wondered what would happen if I really committed. Could I, Sue Reynolds, get into the top twenty-five? Could I become an alternate for Team USA?

I didn't realize it, but I was changing. I had started out as a beginner, hoping to cross the finish line. Then I was a recreational triathlete who trained to set personal bests. I appreciated so many things about recreational triathlon. I loved how people were kind and supportive of one another. And I loved doing the activities that I'd enjoyed as a child—swimming, biking, and running. Now I was transitioning into a competitive triathlete, someone who also found joy in the challenge of racing against others.

But while I found joy in competition, I also found sadness. I had always strived for win-wins, so everyone would be happy. By design, however, competition is a win-lose situation. The winner will be happy; the loser will be sad. I didn't like the idea of someone being sad, and I wondered why I wanted to compete. My self-image didn't depend on athletic performance. I was not a workaholic who felt obligated to train and race. I didn't enjoy dominating people. But something about beating the woman to the bridge at Nationals during the swim made me realize I loved competing. It just didn't make sense. I decided to talk to Coach Brant.

I explained to Coach Brant that I was struggling with the concept of being competitive. I told him how I'd enjoyed beating the woman in Milwaukee to the bridge even though I had shoved her underwater in the process. "I think there may be a monster inside of me," I confided. I just couldn't reconcile the gentle, kind side of me with the competitive monster I had discovered.

Coach Brant listened and then helped me understand that athletic competition is not mean-spirited, spiteful, or hateful. It's a game that involves our bodies, just as checkers is a game that involves our minds. When people play competitive games, everyone knows that someone is going to win and someone is going to lose. Winning and losing do not define who we are; it's just something that happens at one moment in time. Coach Brant pointed out that I wasn't trying to shove that woman underwater. I was simply trying to get to the bridge first. And he added that he knew that if I bumped into someone on the street, I'd step back and say, "Excuse me."

Coach Brant's explanation of competition made sense to me. Just like checkers, triathlon is a game. I could look for win-wins in every other part of my life, but in competitive triathlon, I could seek the win.

With my discomfort about competition resolved, my thoughts returned to Team USA, and again I wondered what would happen if I really committed myself to triathlon. I wondered if I could improve enough to be an alternate for Team USA. I didn't have much confidence in my athletic ability, but I had huge confidence in my tenacity and work ethic.

Having designed and implemented several award-winning programs in the course of my career, I knew the kind of commitment it takes to be a peak performer. That commitment calls for all-in focus on the goal, no excuses, whatever it takes. That commitment doesn't recognize failure as an option. You figure out what needs to be done, and then you do it. If that doesn't work, then you try something else. That kind of commitment had caused me to gain weight as I ate to stay awake during my all-nighters. While I questioned my athletic ability, I never questioned my tenacity. I knew how to be all in.

Secretly, without telling my coach, I decided to go for it. It would be such an honor to be an alternate for Team USA. My first secret goal—walking the 5K—had become transformed into something far beyond what I could ever have imagined. Now I had a new secret goal—to be an alternate for Team USA.

I began by writing the names of the twenty-eight women who finished before me at the USA Triathlon National Championship on a piece of paper, which I posted on my refrigerator. I set my one and only goal for the next twelve months: to work harder than every one of the women on that list. Instead of triathlon working around life, life would now work around triathlon. At the end of one year, when we were all at Nationals again, I would see how many places I could move up the list. If I didn't move up, that would be OK, as long as I knew I had left no stone unturned.

As I started to plan my pathway to becoming a Team USA alternate, I thought about the change formula that I taught leadership teams as part of my work. The formula I use is adapted from work by Kathie Dannemiller and Robert Jacobs.

$$\text{Change occurs when } D \times V \times B \times K > R,$$

where D is dissatisfaction with the current state, V is vision of the desired future state, B is belief in oneself as a change maker, K is knowledge of the first few steps, and R is resistance to change. I understood that becoming an alternate for Team USA would be possible only if all five components of the change formula were in place.

First, I thought about the right side of the equation. For change to occur, I needed to reduce resistance (R) from any source. After thinking at length, I decided the biggest resistance would come from within me in the form of fear. I anticipated being afraid of injury, failure, and what people thought about me. But I also knew how to address resistance; I had my fear boxes that would help me reduce my fears when they emerged.

Then I thought about the left side of the equation. I was dissatisfied (D) with the current state. I didn't want to be in the middle of the pack in my big races. I had a vision (V) of where I wanted to go: I saw myself as an alternate for Team USA. I had belief (B) in myself as a change maker. But one component was missing. I did not have knowledge (K) of the first few steps. When it came to training in a way that would enable me to compete with the best triathletes in the country, I was clueless. I needed to talk to Coach Brant.

When Coach Brant and I met, I didn't share that I hoped to be an alternate for Team USA. Given that I was still really a beginner, I figured he'd think that was silly. So I only told him I wanted to be "among the best triathletes in the country." I remembered how I'd tried to imitate my daughter-in-law's eating habits when I first started losing weight, and now I wanted to emulate the training habits of an elite triathlete. I asked Coach Brant if he could help me understand how elite athletes thought and behaved, and if he could train me as an elite. I thought Coach Brant might laugh or roll his eyes since I was still just a beginner, but to his credit, he agreed. At that moment, we became a team of two with a common mission—training like an elite triathlete.

Training like an elite meant no missed workouts, no excuses, no whining. As we started down that road, I discovered I had become a different person. I no longer asked my husband to put my shoes on my feet in the morning. I no longer believed I didn't deserve water at the aid stations. I no longer avoided looking at myself in the mirror. I was developing confidence. The confidence didn't come from the weight loss or the progress I was making in triathlon. The confidence came from facing and overcoming fears that emerged in unfamiliar and difficult challenges and realizing I had the courage to keep going.

I was a new person, but in a sense, I was a former me. I was the ten-year-old who loved riding her bike, climbing trees, and playing tackle football with kids in the neighborhood. For the first time since I was a child, I felt like I was myself. For the past five decades, the athlete inside me had been hidden, because girls weren't supposed to play sports, because I was supposed to look a certain way and build a certain life, because I didn't know large people could exercise, because I had a list of things I couldn't do, because I was scared. Now the athlete inside me was healthy and active. I knew who I was—who I had always been. I felt at peace. I was an athlete. And although that athlete had been buried for fifty years, I felt so blessed to have discovered the athlete inside at age sixty, when decades of my life lay ahead of me for training and racing.

• • •

Blessed. That was a word I'd never used when I started losing weight. I knew I had a wonderful husband and sons, but God was far from my mind. But as my journey progressed, it became my favorite word.

Chapter 8

I KNOW THIS IS YOU, GOD

A spiritual journey was the furthest thing from my mind when I started dieting and exercising. But when I had lost about ninety pounds, around the time I ran my first 5K, my weight loss started to feel a bit surreal. I'd look at myself in the mirror and shake my head in disbelief. I mean, who loses *ninety* pounds? I had the strangest sense that my journey was happening *to* me rather than because of my actions. It seemed like I was riding a magic carpet, with someone else doing the driving. I was confused. In the very back of my mind, I started to wonder if my weight loss had something to do with God.

I grew up in a Christian family. We went to church every Sunday, but we never read the Bible or talked about our faith as a family. Before dinner, we said a prayer: "Thank you, God, for this food. Bless it to our use and us for thy service. Amen." But that was it. Outside of praying before dinner, we never spoke about God or our faith. While my family didn't pray out loud, I often prayed silently within myself. As a child, those prayers usually involved me asking God for something. "Please, God, let me learn how to ride my bike. Please, God, let me ace this test. Please, God, let me marry the right man." In college, I wasn't inspired by organized religion and stopped attending church, but I kept a journal where I wrote to God about the meaning of life and everything else that confused me. Whenever I faced a practical or ethical question, I discussed it with God in my journal.

My husband also is a Christian. When we first started dating after college, he took me to a church service. After my years of not attending church, it felt wonderful to hear familiar prayers and hymns. I felt at home. We raised both of our sons as Christians, but as in my family, discussions about faith happened only in church. On one occasion, I tried to change that situation. I asked my husband and our sons to share the things for which they were grateful. Then I wrote a family prayer that included each of their words and made copies to read together as a family before dinner. Unfortunately, the prayer was lengthy, and every time I suggested we recite it, I heard, "Oh, mom. Do we have to say *that* prayer?" Twenty years later, our sons still talk about the family prayer, so I know my effort made an impression. At the time, however, prayer as a family was not going to happen. Instead, I continued to pray my silent prayers with God on a daily basis and in church each weekend.

A few years before I started losing weight, I experienced a strong season of doubt that began with a friend and I having conversations about faith. As we drove to various meetings across the state we explained our views to each other. I shared that I believed in God and was a follower of Jesus. He was an atheist, and as I talked about my Christian beliefs, he presented logical, scientific

explanations that contradicted the existence of God. He wasn't trying to make me into a nonbeliever; he was just presenting his beliefs
as I presented mine.

I wasn't sure how to explain my belief in God. I finally said, "See
that Coke can? It exists, right? How do you know that it exists? You
can see it. You can feel it. That's how it is for me with God. I can
sense God's existence. He just is." I never thought a Coke can would
help me explain God's existence, but I needed something concrete,
and there it was. The can existed; God existed. To me, each was as
concrete as the other.

Our discussions made me think about how to actually know
if God exists. Maybe there were ways of knowing that something
exists besides scientific proof. I thought about beauty as a language
that conveys things that science cannot—sunrises, paintings, and
especially music. I loved to let the music at church wash over me as
the congregation sang in unison. God seemed to be wrapping me in
divine warmth in those moments. But the more I talked to my atheist
friend, the more my faith started to fade.

Over time, I realized how far my faith had fallen and didn't like
what was happening. I still believed in God and went to church
every weekend, but I stopped praying daily and started hiding my
Christianity in fear that I would be judged by others. Worst of all, I
stopped hearing God's words during scripture readings and sermons
at church. Instead, I heard my atheist friend's scientific explanations
regarding stories in the Bible. I started seriously doubting my faith.
Maybe God really was just something people all over the world made
up because they feared death. Maybe core convictions like love and
peace were passed on from one generation to another because they
helped people avoid and resolve conflicts. Doubts raced through my
mind each time I listened to scripture in church.

Then one day, I had had enough. Just as I had done with eating, I said, "Enough," to my doubts about God, and I decided to change. I *did* believe in God. I *wanted* to live as a Christian. I vowed to have the courage to stand tall for my faith and all the things that went with it—the gifts of love, joy, kindness, and peace. It didn't matter to me that I couldn't use science to prove the existence of God. In my heart I knew, and I wanted to return to living with that belief as a part of my daily life.

• • •

The spiritual trip back to God was difficult, but I found God waiting with open arms. Someone once told me that when people return to God, God rejoices with back flips. I hoped God, Jesus, and the Holy Spirit were all doing back flips as I returned to being a more active participant in my faith.

My first step in my journey was to purchase a cross necklace as a symbol of my faith. It took several months to muster up the courage to go into a jewelry store to shop for a cross. I didn't tell anyone what I was doing. My faith had always been private, and I didn't want to announce it to the world. Then it took several more months to find just the right one—a cross that no one would see but I would know was there. I finally found a small gold disk hanging on a thin gold chain. From a distance, it just looked like a little disk. But up close, you could see miniature diamonds forming the shape of a cross. I wore that tiny disk beneath my clothes where no one could see it, but I knew it was there, and it reminded me to be strong.

As I continued moving forward in my triathlon journey, faith continued to become a stronger presence in my life. Our older son (who would later become a pastor) started talking to me about God.

The discussion was awkward at first. He pointed out that our family never talked about God and told me that faith had become an important part of his life that he wanted to share with me. He spoke of the joy that comes with believing and told me that God loves me. He started quoting the Bible all the time. I felt a little bombarded with scripture. I didn't know the Bible well enough to be able to participate in that part of our conversation, and I felt intimidated. But after each talk, I'd think about my son's words and the verses he quoted. With time, they became comfortable to me.

One of the most pivotal moments in my faith journey happened right after the USA Triathlon National Championship. In an email, I told Coach Brant that I had been afraid of letting people down. He responded, "As far as disappointing people, forget that altogether, Sue. It doesn't matter what 'others' think. If we go through life worrying about others, we will never accomplish anything, and we will always feel like we don't measure up. You're perfect the way God made you. Enjoy what he's allowing you to do. He's your only judge, and He loves you regardless."

When I read Coach Brant's words, I felt as though I had been hit in the head with a two-by-four. It was as though the sky had opened, and God was saying, "Listen to me. I am talking to you. I am reaching out to you." I froze. And then I said to myself, *Whoa! What just happened?* First my son talking about God's love, and then my coach, who I hadn't even known was a Christian. That was powerful.

Several days later, during a coached workout at our YMCA, I mustered up the courage to ask Coach Brant about his statement. As we sat on workout mats, he talked quietly about his faith. Talking out loud about God was so new to me, I wasn't sure what words to use. I continued to ask Coach Brant questions about his faith, specifically about the Bible. How often did he read the Bible? How did he memorize all those verses? Coach Brant was patient and nurturing. It seemed strange to be seeking spiritual guidance from a person who was younger than my sons. I told Coach Brant that he should be a pastor. He responded that we are all called to preach in our daily lives, and he explained that coaching was the vehicle that God had given him so he could be available if and when others were ready to talk about God.

Discussions about spirituality are not always easy. During one discussion about salvation with Coach Brant, we struggled to understand each other's beliefs, and we each turned to our clergy for guidance. Coach Brant wrote to me, "These conversations end many relationships. I'm glad we have a relationship that can stand the hard stuff. Even if we don't end up seeing eye to eye, being able to work through this conversation is something most people in the world can't do. Thank you for being willing to work through it."

• • •

As my conversations about faith continued with my son and coach, I started having a stronger and stronger sense that God had something to do with my weight loss and fitness journey. But why? What did God want me to do? And why me? I asked God, "What do you want me to do with these gifts?"

God didn't speak out loud to me, but I sensed God's answer was "These gifts are just for you." That seemed selfish to me. My church taught that we should use our gifts to serve others. I wondered if God wanted me to start a nonprofit to help people lose weight or gain fitness. Over and over, I prayed and asked what God wanted but kept sensing the same response: "These gifts are just for you."

And then one morning in church, it all made sense. Our pastor explained that God actively reaches out to each of us, and one of the ways God does this is through gifts. A light bulb lit up in my head. That was it. God was reaching out to me, seeking my attention. Whoa! God wanted *my* attention. I felt little and big at the same time. I was humbled that God saw enough value in me to reach out to me, but I also felt undeserving of God's attention. Mostly, I felt incredibly loved. Even though I had doubted God's existence and stopped praying, God wanted to have a relationship with me. God was calling *me*.

The blessings that God showered upon me were piling up: my fitness; the joy of swimming, biking, and running; the happiness I felt during triathlons; stronger relationships with my husband and sons. I realized I had been taking other gifts for granted—most notably, having the freedom to pursue my dreams.

Women in other parts of the world, like my friend Salome Kanini (Sally), struggle to be able to participate in the sports they love. Sally, who lives in Nairobi, and I started sending messages back and forth on Facebook after I learned about her efforts to organize the first bike ride for women in Kenya. She explained that in the Kenyan culture, cycling is not considered "ladylike" and is frowned upon for women and girls. Boys can ride a bike to school, but girls have to walk. Men can commute by bike to work, but women do not have that means of transportation. I did a little research online and found that some Kenyan schools had even refused to accept donated bikes because the gift stipulated that a percentage of the bikes had to go to girls. In an area where many people depend on walking, a bike can make a huge difference. Therefore, by getting women involved in cycling events, Sally is a pioneer striving to change a culture for the benefit of others.

Sally named the women's ride Dada (Swahili for "sister") Ride. She not only had to organize the event, but also had to find bikes and helmets for the women and teach them how to ride bikes, since they had not learned how to ride a bike as children. The first Dada Ride was a huge success. It soon evolved into monthly Dada Rides. Then Dada Rides became a registered nongovernmental, nonprofit, and nonpolitical organization with the mission of promoting women and girl's participation in cycling for healthy lifestyles. In addition to the monthly rides, Dada Rides now offers classes in bike maintenance and bike races for women. I deeply admire Sally's courage and commitment to her dreams, as well as the gifts she has given to the women around her.

Of the gifts I have received, the one that most touched me was the kindness that people have showered upon me since the very first steps in my fitness journey. Many, many people encouraged and supported me throughout my weight loss, fitness, and now spiritual journeys when times were tough. Over and over, I experienced kindness that brought tears to my eyes, often from perfect strangers who showed up at just the right moment and said just the right thing to keep me moving forward. Then they disappeared.

The first stranger who showered me with kindness was a woman who passed me on her bike almost every day when I first started running at 280 pounds. Each time she passed, she gave me a big smile and shouted, "Lookin' good!" At 280 pounds, I was pretty sure that I was not "lookin' good." I was fully aware of my bouncing belly as I ran down the road, and I was sure that my gait looked more like a shuffle than a run. But her words boosted my confidence. Each time I ran, I hoped to see her. I never learned her name. I never spoke to her. She will never know the impact she had on my life.

The blessing of kindness entered my life again at the start of the OneAmerica 500 Festival Mini-Marathon. When I approached the start line at 190 pounds, I found thirty-four thousand people waiting for the race to begin. Their brightly colored T-shirts and jackets bounced as they jumped up and down, waiting nervously for the race to start. Each runner stood in a corral created by ropes that stretched across the road to separate the runners by anticipated finish times. The fastest runners were in the first corral. I was assigned to a corral in the back, right in front of the "cleanup bus." That bus would travel at the slowest pace a person could run and still make the race's cut-off time. If you couldn't keep in front of the bus, the officials would make you board the bus and ride back to the race start.

I literally had nightmares about staying in front of that bus. In my nightmare, the bus was an angry monster with a huge mouth. It chased the slower runners, and I was one of them. I ran as fast as I could but was losing ground. I feared being eaten and then sitting in the bus with my head hung in shame as it drove me back to the race start.

I found my corral in front of the bus, but there was no room inside the roped-off space. People were literally shoulder to shoulder without an inch between them. I stared helplessly at the mass of people. How was I going to squeeze in? Suddenly, a path seemed to appear among the people, leading to a man in a white shirt and white cap. He was motioning for me to join him. I ducked under the rope and stood by his side.

My nerves began getting the best of me, and I was fighting tears. I had only run 9 miles in training. Coach Brant assured me that my total weekly miles and the excitement of being close to the finish line would carry me the last 4 miles, but I was not sure I could make the half-marathon's 13.1 miles. On the verge of a meltdown, I started chatting with the man in the white cap. He was kind. He told me that science had proven that runners are capable of covering three times their longest distance in training. I did the math. Three times 9 miles equaled 27 miles. Then 13.1 miles should be doable. His words filled me with confidence. I started to feel calm. I would make it.

Just before the start, he assured me that everything would be fine. When I turned to thank him for his kindness, he was gone. I skimmed the crowd, looking for his white cap. No white cap. He had disappeared. Like the woman on the bike, he would never know the impact he'd had on my life.

The most amazing kindness came later in my journey from a man that I met in Clermont, Florida, a few days before a triathlon I raced there in my third season. When my husband and I arrived in Clermont, we drove straight to the beach at Lake Louisa, so I could do a swim workout prior to checking into our hotel. My husband stayed in the parking lot to guard my bike, which was on the back of our car. I walked alone on a boardwalk through a swampy area of cypress trees and came upon a beach that was completely deserted—no lifeguard, no sunbathers, no picnickers, no children, no boats. Not a person was in sight. The water, stained by cypress trees, was the color of Coca-Cola. And then I saw a sign that said, "Beware of alligators."

I stood under a clear sky on the deserted beach and thought about swimming in a lake with alligators. I knew they would be more scared of me than I was of them, but I worried that I'd step on one or get between a mama alligator and her baby. I knew that this fear belonged in the Do Not Think about These Things box, but I couldn't get past it. I had not missed a workout in two years, but swimming with alligators at a deserted beach was not going to happen. No way. I went into the bathhouse with my head hung low and changed into my swimsuit, although I was sure that I was not getting in the water.

When I came out, I was surprised to see a white speedboat sitting on the sand. I hadn't heard it pull up. A man and a woman were gazing at the sparkling water of the deserted lake. As we chatted, I explained that I needed to do a swim workout in preparation for my race, but I was afraid to go in the water because of the alligators. The man said, "I'll protect you from the alligators." He explained that he'd grown up in the area and was not afraid of alligators. "I'm going to stand in the water while you swim. I'll watch for alligators, and if I see any, I'll scare them away." Then he walked into the lake until he was standing in chest-deep water where the marshy grass stopped growing.

Cautiously, I swam back and forth across the open water. Every time I took a breath, I could see the man scanning the water, looking for alligators. He stood in the lake for my entire swim workout. Later, his wife told me that she had experienced a spiritual aha moment in her life, and he had been a big part of it. I don't know their names. I will probably never see them again. Like the woman on the bike and the man at the half marathon, they will never know the impact of their kindness.

Through these experiences and many others, I began to learn about the power of kindness. I started to understand that two words or some other small act of kindness can make a huge difference, can change a life. The amount of kindness that was being showered on me felt surreal. It was raining kindness. I started wondering who all these kind people were.

I brought this question to Bob, the man who'd set up Brian and me on our first date. Bob had recently become a Christian deacon. Over lunch with Brian, Bob, and Bob's wife, I shyly told Bob through tears about my weight loss and fitness journeys and all the kind strangers who kept popping into my life. I asked if they were angels. He just smiled. As we were saying good-bye, he told me, "Keep seeing the face of God in others." A light bulb went off in my head. These kind people were the face of God.

With that new understanding, I began seeing God's love in people's words and actions all around me. God was everywhere. I found myself looking up from time to time and quietly whispering words that a new friend had shared with me: "I know this is you, God. Thank you." I also began realizing that God's love can flow from me to others, too. I hid two small decals on my bike. One read, "Go with God." The other said, "Let your light shine."

I decided that while God's gifts of weight loss and fitness were "just for me," I wanted to use those gifts to do good deeds, to help others, and to be the face of God for others like the woman on the bike had been for me. I hoped that through small acts of everyday kindness and by sharing my story, I might help others move forward with a change they wanted to make in their life, whatever that change might be.

As the spiritual side of my journey was unfolding, I kept training and preparing for races. The World Triathlon Series race in Chicago and the USA Triathlon National Championship in Milwaukee were major turning points for me. Having determined that I was near the middle of the pack among women my age, I looked forward with excitement to training as an elite triathlete in preparation for the next season. I wondered how far I could go.

TRIATHLON SEASON 3

DEVELOPING GRIT

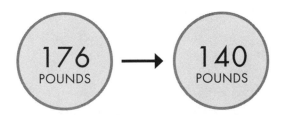

176 POUNDS → 140 POUNDS

Chapter 9

NO STONE UNTURNED

C oach Brant and I sat down in September to map out my training for the fall, winter, and spring as I prepared for my third
triathlon season. This year would be different: I would be training as
an elite, even though, with just two seasons of triathlon experience, I
still considered myself a beginner.

I had already made some changes to my routine that I knew were
more aligned with an elite performer's mind-sets and behaviors.
Most notably, I adopted a "no stone unturned" approach to my triathlon preparation. My self-imposed rule required me to implement
anything I could think of that would make me faster, no matter how
big or small, difficult, or boring. I also committed to my favorite
mantra, "No excuses, whatever it takes, find a way." And finally, I
pledged to not see roadblocks as dead ends. Instead, I would see

them as temporary detours or bumps in the road, and figure out a way through or around them. Nothing would stop me.

I also started seeking role models, and had many. I admired some of the coaches I heard on podcasts, including Matt Dixon, Adam Zucco, and Suzanne Atkinson. They not only talked about the nuts and bolts of triathlon, but also discussed the mental aspects of performing at a high level. I loved listening to their inspiring ideas as I ran.

However, the person I looked up to the most was Gwen Jorgensen, the first Olympic champion in triathlon from the United States. I loved watching her compete at the World Triathlon Series in Chicago. I highly respected her method for setting goals, her work ethic, and her hunger for success. In addition, Gwen carried herself with a humility that I admired. Throughout the year, when I wasn't sure how to handle a situation, I'd ask myself, *What would Gwen do?*

I had confidence in my ability to handle the mental side of training as an elite, but I depended on Coach Brant to teach me how to physically train as an elite triathlete. My education began when we met in September. The first thing he explained was how to approach A, B, and C races. I would have one A race: the USA Triathlon National Championship in August. In that race, our goal was to place as high as I possibly could. We'd use all my other races to test different pacing strategies and teach me how to race. Some of those races would be B races. Those were races where we wanted to do well and therefore would rest my body slightly before the race. But most of my races would be local C races, where we would treat the race as though it was just another day of training.

Next, Coach Brant explained how the year would be laid out. We'd spend months building a base by doing long distances at a relatively relaxed pace. That base would prepare my body for the

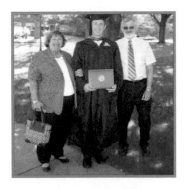

Our son's graduation from graduate school when I weighed 335 pounds. This is one of the few photos I have of myself as a heavier person.

My "before" photo on the first day of Meltdown Bootcamp. The size of my belly made it impossible to do everyday tasks like tie my shoes or fit in a restaurant booth.

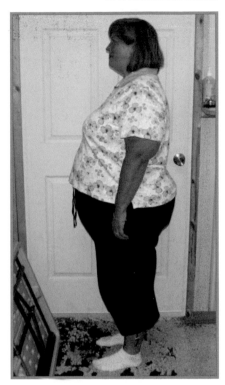

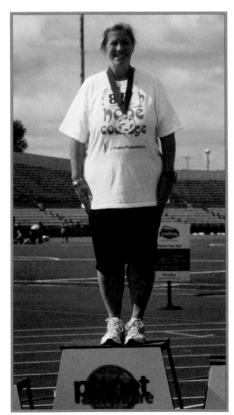

SEASON 1: Walking into transition after the bike segment at my first triathlon. I conquered many fears to get to this point!

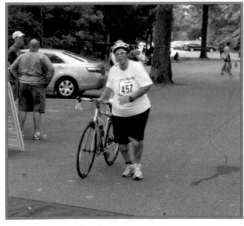

SEASON 1: My first time standing on a podium. I always wore this t-shirt for inspiration at races. The front said, "Strength. Hope. Courage."

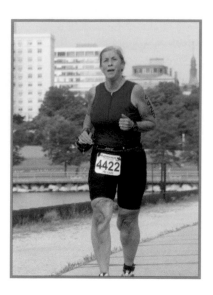

SEASON 2: My first USA Triathlon National Championship. My goal in Milwaukee was to make it across the finish line. PHOTO BY: FinisherPix®

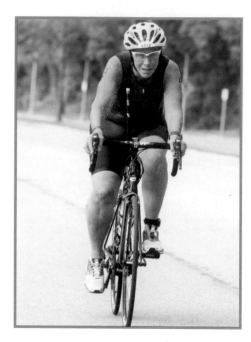

SEASON 2: Before Nationals, I purchased a competitive bike, but I was still too scared to use aerobars or clip-in pedals. PHOTO BY: FinisherPix®

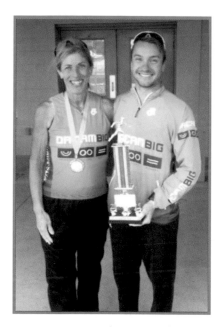

SEASON 3: Coach Brant and I sometimes competed in the same races. In this race, he was top male for all age groups, while I was first female in my age group.

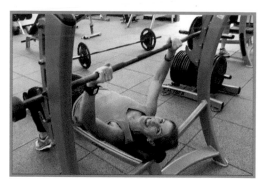

SEASON 3: Although I still considered myself to be a beginner, I asked Coach Brant to train me like an elite triathlete. That meant doing whatever it took to be faster, including lifting weights.

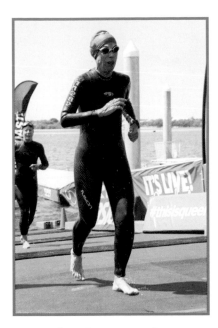

SEASON 3: Part of being fast is finding "free speed." A new bike with aerobars and wide-rimmed wheels made me more aerodynamic. To save time, I mounted my bike barefoot and then slipped into shoes that were clipped to my pedals while the bike was rolling. PHOTO BY: FinisherPix®

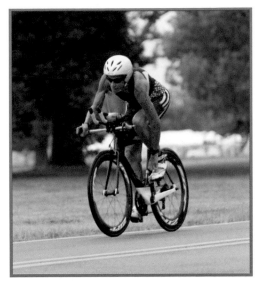

Running from the water to the transition area where I will jump on my bike. Along the way, I'll strip off my wet suit as I run to save time. PHOTO BY: FinisherPix®

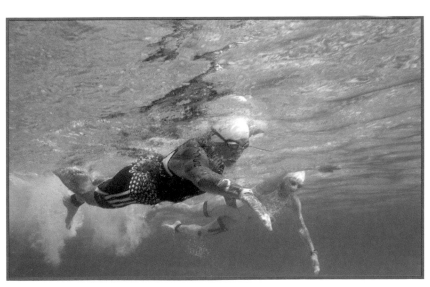

SEASON 4: My first Worlds! When I glanced at the woman next to me during the swim and saw she wore a Mexico uniform, I got a little choked up. I couldn't believe I was racing on behalf of the USA at Worlds. PHOTO BY: 2DIGITAL

SEASON 4: Exiting the water at Worlds in Cozumel. I didn't know until after the race that a rogue ocean current had made the swim more challenging. PHOTO BY: 2DIGITAL

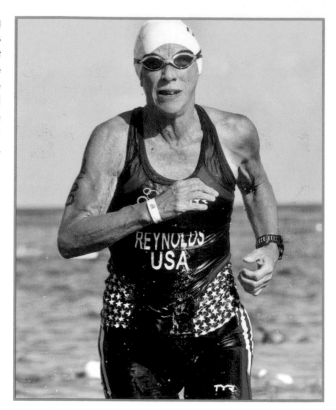

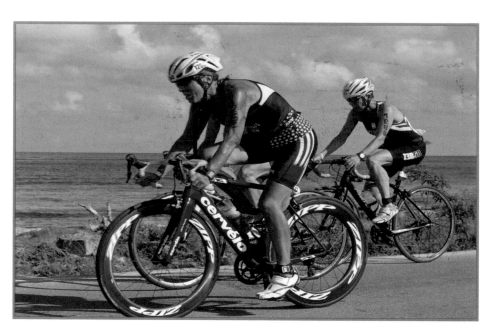

SEASON 4: For the first time ever, the bike segment at Worlds was draft legal. While I had been scared to ride in this new format, I loved riding with a pack of bikes, and ended up with the fastest bike split among all countries! PHOTO BY: 2DIGITAL

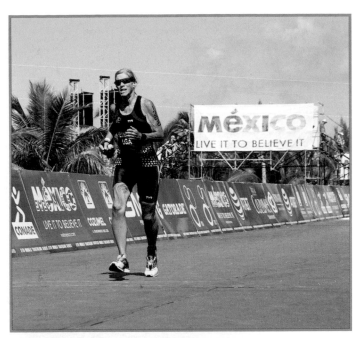

SEASON 4: Running down the finish chute at Worlds in Cozumel in incredible heat. After giving all I had to the race, I hoped I had enough gas in the tank to get over the finish line. PHOTO BY: 2DIGITAL

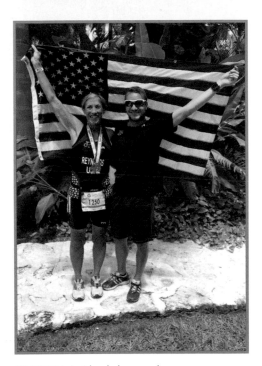

SEASON 4: Posing with my husband, Brian, after my first Worlds. God answered my prayers when he sent Brian into my life. I've been married to my best friend for over forty years.

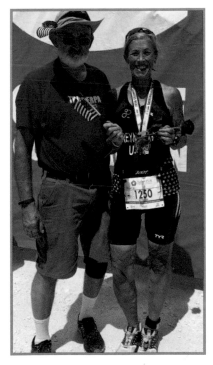

SEASON 4: I had dreamed for years about posing with the American flag after Worlds. Such a joy to hold up the flag with Coach Brant.

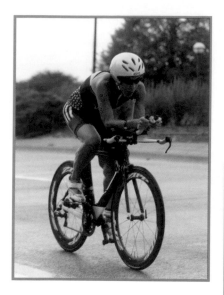

SEASON 5: Racing in Omaha, Nebraska at the USAT National Championship, and trying to be as aero as possible. PHOTO BY: FinisherPix®

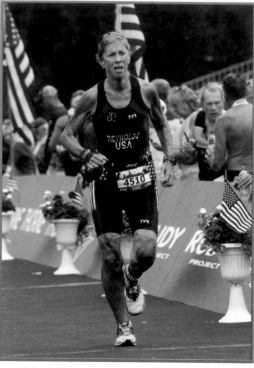

SEASON 5: Racing to the finish line at the USA Triathlon National Championship in Omaha. Hoping to qualify for Team USA—and I did! PHOTO BY: FinisherPix®

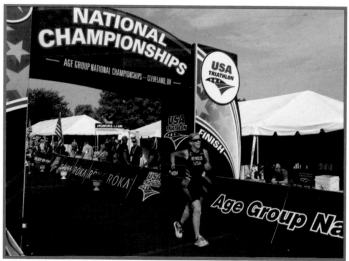

SEASON 5: Crossing the finish line at Nationals. Some people raise their arms in celebration with a big smile as they cross the finish line. I always look like I'm ready to die. PHOTO BY: FinisherPix®

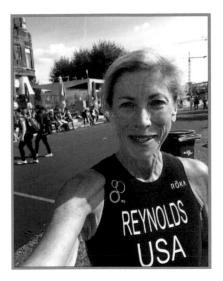

SEASON 5: Race morning at my second Worlds in Rotterdam, Netherlands. Super pumped!

SEASON 5: Halfway through the run at Worlds in Rotterdam. I'm working to execute Coach Brant's race plan perfectly. PHOTO BY: FinisherPix®

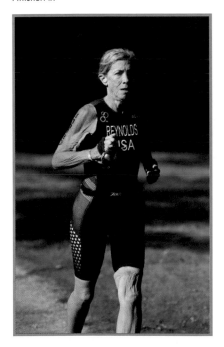

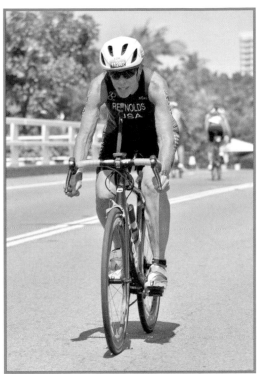

Triathlon bikes with aerobars are illegal in draft-legal races, so when racing at Worlds, I ride my road bike. PHOTO BY: FinisherPix®

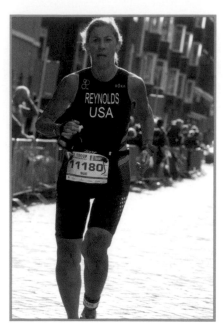

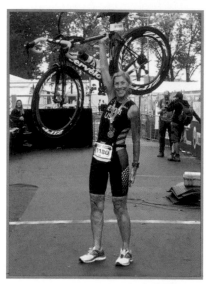

SEASON 5: I did it! Sixth place finish (and first American) at Worlds! I'm thrilled with the outcome, but more pleased that I worked hard all year and executed my race plan well. I love this photo. It shows every bit of the joy I was feeling at the end of the race.

SEASON 5: I'm approaching the finish chute at my second Worlds. After swimming, biking, and running, every ounce of my being is focused on keeping my feet moving as I push for a strong finish. PHOTO BY: FinisherPix®

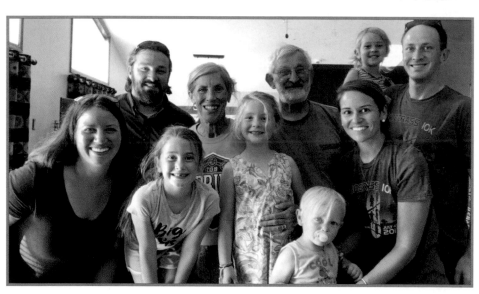

My triathlon journey wouldn't have been possible without the love and support from my family. Clockwise from top right: My younger son, Andy (holding Caroline). The rest of Andy's family—Laura, Mack, Emma Kate, and Harper. My older son's wife, Megan, followed by my older son, Mike. Me. My hubby and best friend, Brian.

hard work that Coach Brant would give me later. Every fourth week, I'd have a recovery week, when the work would be very light. Coach Brant explained that recovery weeks were key to my training. During that time, that my body would rebuild itself into a stronger and faster body.

After the base phase, we'd begin a series of three-week builds that would include intervals, which involve covering short distances at high intensity with short rests in between. Again, we'd take every fourth week as a recovery week. Then, three weeks prior to my A race, we'd have two peak weeks. Those weeks would push my body to the max and result in the biggest gains in fitness. Finally, a few days before my A race, we'd taper. Tapering would allow my body to rest. I'd lose some fitness during those days, but I'd also lose fatigue. The idea was to get to the start line with the most fitness and the least fatigue. That made sense to me. I was all in.

Finally, Coach Brant talked about two other sides of training. First was strength training. The idea of lifting weights at age sixty-two seemed a little silly. Imagining myself in the weight room with all the young athletes, I was amused. But if that's what needed to be done, then I would do it. No stone unturned. Coach Brant also talked about sleep. He would begin monitoring my sleep daily. That freaked me out a little; Coach Brant was monitoring every minute of my life. But again, if that's what it took to train as an elite, then so be it.

I didn't talk to Coach Brant about my weight, but I knew that was part of the equation, too. When we first started working together, I told Coach Brant that I didn't want to discuss how much I weighed. I feared that Coach Brant would start to sound like my mother, and I'd begin hiding peanut butter and jelly sandwiches to eat in secret. Coach Brant understood. His respect for my request increased my trust in him.

• • •

After our talk about my annual training plan, I began thinking more about my secret goal. Striving to be an alternate for Team USA in three years after weighing 335 pounds seemed a little crazy. But then again, I knew there was a place for crazy goals.

A few months earlier, I'd heard Mark Allen speak. Mark and Dave Scott are tied for the most Ironman World Championships at six apiece. In Ironman-distance triathlons, people swim for 2.4 miles, bike for 112 miles, and then run for 26.2 miles. To be world champion six times was amazing. During Mark's remarks, he talked about three kinds of goals: crazy, realistic, and fallback. His crazy goals were secrets, because they were so outrageous, people would think he was nuts if he shared them. My goal to be an alternate for Team USA in three years was my crazy goal, and like Mark, I kept it a secret, even from Coach Brant.

Mark's realistic goals were ones he felt he could reach with hard work, like completing a race within a certain time period. On off days, when he couldn't reach his realistic goals, he quickly set fallback goals. I set realistic goals every day in training to complete intervals in the time designated by Coach Brant. His targets for the hardest intervals were always perfectly placed. I could reach them, but only if I put in max effort. But sometimes I just had an off day and came up short over and over. On days when I couldn't hit the target, I quickly set a fallback goal and strived to reach that.

Gwen Jorgensen's approach to goal setting also spoke to me. In a Facebook post exactly one year prior to her Olympic win, she wrote, "I believe in process-driven goals, but I still aspire for a golden outcome." Gwen helped me understand the difference between process goals and outcome goals. Process goals are things you control every day to support the desired outcome. My biggest process goal was to do *exactly* what Coach Brant told me to do every day (no excuses, whatever it takes, find a way). While I worked toward my process goals, I aspired for my golden outcome—to become an alternate for Team USA in three years.

I liked process goals because they were within my control, and I could guarantee that they would be met. In contrast, outcome goals were out of my control. While I could control my effort, I couldn't control what kind of weather we had, who else showed up to compete, what kind of day they had, if I got boxed in during the swim, or whether I rode my bike over a tack and got a flat tire. So I focused on meeting my process goal by doing everything that Coach Brant told me to do—no exceptions. I knew that if I met all of my process goals, I was more likely to reach my outcome goal, and at the finish line, I could hold my head high, regardless of the race results.

Some triathlon coaches touch base with their athletes every day, and I asked Coach Brant if he would create a new coaching package that included daily narratives from me with feedback from him each evening. He agreed. This daily accountability system was even closer to the one I had experienced in Meltdown Bootcamp. But it was more than just accountability. Every day in my narrative, I'd ask Coach Brant questions about training, my data, or my technique, and each evening, he answered those questions. I had my own private triathlon tutor.

This level of training quickly took over my free time. Getting my gear ready, stretching, training, showering, studying my data, and sending feedback to Coach Brant took four to five hours each day. Triathletes with children tend to get up early in the morning to train before getting their kids ready for school. But my sons were grown, and I never liked getting out of bed in the morning, so I trained after work, had a late dinner, and then packed my workout gear for the next day.

Luckily, Brian was patient when training made me too tired to have conversations in the evening. But every Sunday, my rest day, we'd go to church and then out to lunch. Having that time for us was important. On race day, too, Brian had valuable roles: He carried my gear, pulling a wagon that held all my swim, bike, and run gear. He served as my timekeeper, making sure I was on schedule as I set up in transition and did my warm-up. Brian learned the routine and let me know if I forgot to do something. Finally, he functioned as my videographer, providing videos for Coach Brant and me to analyze after the race. On race day, my coach, husband, and I were a team of three.

Sometimes, when I had to work late, my training got pushed back to ten o'clock in the evening or later. If it was too dark to train outside, I'd ride on a stationary bike or run on a treadmill in the basement. Finally, Coach Brant asked me to start training in the morning so I could train with a fresh body. He explained that my body was tired after working all day in the office and would do better earlier in the day. Immediately, I thought of my commitment to leave no stone unturned. If training in the morning would make me faster, then that's what I needed to do. I talked to my work colleagues, explained the situation, and asked what they thought of me working between noon and eight in the evening. With their agreement, I started training in the mornings.

Slowly, my life was changing. Instead of triathlon fitting around my life, my life now fit around triathlon. I was training like an elite triathlete. Secretly, I wondered where that would take me. Would I be an alternate for Team USA in three years?

Even though I was training like an elite triathlete, it was difficult at times to think of myself as an athlete at all. After sitting on the couch for decades as an obese person, it seemed ridiculous that I could be an athlete. Calling myself an athlete felt silly; instead, I'd refer to myself as a pseudo-athlete or an athlete-wannabe. Coach Brant would correct me. He'd tell me that I had athletic goals, trained every day, and had a coach. That made me an athlete. Still, I struggled to feel comfortable with thinking of myself as an athlete.

During one of our winter sit-down meetings, Coach Brant took our conversation in a surprising direction. He opened by saying, "Sue, you need to develop swag." I must have looked puzzled, because he went on to say, "Sue, you are good. You need to start thinking of yourself as a top athlete, because you are. You have the potential to go far. You need to carry yourself with swag, because you are good, really good."

His comments blew me away. He not only talked about me being an athlete, but also talked about my potential as an athlete at the top of her sport. I wasn't sure what "swag" meant. When I thought of swag, I pictured a self-consumed person covered with muscles and an immense ego who boasted about athletic accomplishments. That certainly didn't fit how I saw myself. Coach Brant explained that swag is not something you put on. It just comes naturally as you developed confidence. He said true swag is never purposeful or boastful. It just happens as personal confidence grows. I understood what Coach Brant was saying. He didn't want me to strut around like a prima donna. He wanted me to develop confidence and to carry myself with confidence.

I felt a small fire ignite inside me when I thought about Coach Brant's words. He thought I was good—really, really good. He thought I had potential. He believed I could go far. I let those words soak in and felt excitement begin to form. Coach Brant believed in me. I was starting to believe in myself.

Our sit-down meetings became more frequent. Usually, I'd come with a list of questions about technique or training. But sometimes we'd talk about a fear that was interfering with my training. At one meeting, Coach Brant told me that he could tell something had been bothering me for several days. I didn't want to share my fear with him, but I knew being open would help Coach Brant be the best coach he could be. Finally, after mustering courage, I told him that I thought I had disappointed him and feared he didn't want to coach me anymore.

Coach Brant's response was perfect. First, he told me that it wasn't true. I had not disappointed him, and he did want to coach me. Then he explained that we needed to keep our coach-athlete relationship open and honest, so it could be a productive relationship. He instructed me to tell him immediately whenever something was bothering me, not to hold it inside for days. That is something I have aspired to do ever since. It's not always easy, but Coach Brant is always receptive, and the result of sharing what I think has always been positive. The trust between us continues to grow.

A short while later, I shared my secret goal with Coach Brant. I told him I wanted to work hard for three years and become an alternate for Team USA at the end of that period. Coach Brant replied, "Let's not be an alternate. Let's make the team outright, and let's do it *this* year!"

I just stared. I could not imagine that he was serious. But he was serious, and he was pumped. His contagious excitement spread quickly. The more excited he seemed, the more excited I felt. Suddenly, my "crazy" goal turned into a "realistic" goal, and my three-year timeline turned into right now. Unbelievable! With great excitement, I pledged myself to doing whatever it took to earn a position on Team USA during the coming season.

Coach Brant never said so, but I imagined that one of his coaching goals was to take an athlete to Team USA and the Triathlon Age Group World Championship. It was a win-win. We both wanted the same outcome, and we were journeying toward a common goal together. I began to see that Coach Brant's work ethic was just like mine. We were both all in, whatever it took. We were partners with distinct roles. He was the brain who would write the perfect training plan. I was the executor who would implement that plan perfectly. What made our partnership special was that even more than we cared about our own dream, we cared about the other's dream. We each had two reasons for working hard: for our self and for the other.

Just after Christmas, I mentioned to Coach Brant that Brian and I were planning to take a vacation in Florida, and I asked what he thought. "In terms of training," he responded, "you're better off staying home, where you can do sound workouts every day." I was torn. I wanted to have a vacation, but if we went to Florida, I knew that when I crossed the finish line, I'd be wondering what would have happened if I had trained at home. I also knew that if I made this one exception to my no-stone-unturned approach, it would be easier to make a second exception, and then a third. I talked with Brian, but we didn't need to discuss much. He understood that being all in means being all in. We canceled our vacation plans so I could train at home. Life truly revolved around triathlon.

In the spring, Coach Brant and I received disturbing news about the Triathlon Age Group World Championship, where I would compete if I qualified for Team USA during the USA Triathlon National Championship. The International Triathlon Union announced that the sprint distance at Worlds would now include a draft-legal bike portion. "Draft-legal" means bikes would be allowed to form groups where riders would position themselves a few inches behind the bike in front of them, hoping to benefit from a draft, as the racers do in the Tour de France. Riding bikes that close together greatly increases the potential for crashes. If a bike goes down in front, everyone behind that bike is likely to go down, too. Because of the danger, drafting in triathlons is illegal in almost all triathlons in the United States; bikes must stay twenty-three feet away from each other, except when passing.

I wasn't sure I wanted to be on Team USA if that meant I would compete in a draft-legal race at Worlds. I had two options: I could continue to seek a position on Team USA to compete at my sprint distance, knowing that I would compete in a draft-legal race at Worlds if I qualified, or I could try to qualify for Team USA in the longer, standard distance, which was to remain a nondraft race at Worlds.

Coach Brant had mixed feelings. He didn't want to give up on the dream of competing at the sprint distance at Worlds just because of the challenging new format. He also pointed out that all the training I had been doing was designed to prepare me for racing at the sprint distance. On the other hand, he was also concerned about my safety in the new draft-legal format. Both of us were torn.

Before making a final decision, I asked everyone I could for advice. With one exception, everyone told me to stay away from draft-legal races because they were dangerous. But one person, Adam Zucco, a triathlon coach and the host of one of my favorite podcasts, Superfly Coaching Podcast, had a different opinion. In response to an email I sent him to ask his thoughts about draft-legal triathlons, he wrote, "I say you pursue your passion, why not? . . . What's the worst that could happen? You decide it's not for you and you let the pack go? I think that's a reasonable risk. It's not like you are forced to ride in a huge pack." That made sense to me. This was my passion, and I could adjust during the race if the situation felt dangerous by pulling back and letting the pack of bikes go ahead. I called Coach Brant, shared Adam's thoughts, and said, "Let's do this!"

We then received more disturbing news. USA Triathlon, the governing body for triathlon in the United States, decided to change its qualification criteria for Team USA and the world championship. Instead of eighteen people qualifying at Nationals, only eight would qualify. I was devastated. Going from twenty-ninth to eighth felt impossible. When I explained the situation to Coach Brant, he responded with a smile, "Then let's be eighth!" He wasn't giving up on the dream, and he didn't want me to give up either.

The pressure of such a huge goal—rising from twenty-ninth to eighth in one year—felt immense. I was afraid that I'd let down Coach Brant. I continued to train and meet all of my process goals, but some of the joy had gone away. The thought of Coach Brant being disappointed if I didn't finish in the top eight lay heavily on my spirit. I knew I had to talk to Coach Brant about the situation.

Finally, at the pool one day, I told Coach Brant that I felt intense pressure and explained that the thought of disappointing him made me miserable and took the joy out of training. I talked about Gwen Jorgensen's process goals and outcome goals and asked if we could focus on our process goals and take joy in whatever the outcome might be. Coach Brant understood, but he was also honest. He told me that he hoped I would make Team USA, and if that didn't happen, he would be disappointed.

It took me a long time to understand what Coach Brant was saying. But then it made sense to me: when you work hard to reach a goal and miss it, it just makes sense that you're disappointed you didn't reach your goal. That's just part of racing. At the same time, you can find deep satisfaction in knowing you did everything you could to reach your goal. The more I thought about it, the more I realized that's how I felt, too. I would be disappointed if I didn't finish in the top eight, but at the same time, I would know that I had given everything I had every day as we prepared, and I would feel immensely satisfied with my performance. If we missed the top eight, we would not wallow in that disappointment. We would celebrate all that we had accomplished throughout the year and make plans to move forward with another attempt a year later.

Then, a few weeks later, USA Triathlon announced they were sponsoring a new draft-legal sprint triathlon to be held in November, and an additional ten people would qualify for Team USA at that race. If I didn't finish in the top eight at Nationals, I could travel to Florida in November to race in the Draft-Legal Triathlon World Qualifier race. We formed a new plan that I would first try to qualify by placing in the top eight at Nationals. If that didn't happen, I'd attempt to qualify in the top ten at the Draft-Legal Triathlon World Qualifier. Either way, I'd be a member of Team USA.

As summer approached, my training transitioned from base phase to build phase, and the workouts became incredibly hard. Coach Brant often assigned a series of intervals at max effort with very little rest in between. In swim workouts, the rests were often only ten seconds. I had enough time to inhale quickly four times, and then I'd have to push off the wall again with my heart still racing from the previous interval. I began turning swim intervals into a game called Hit-the-Target, and I'd challenge myself to nail each interval. Despite my best efforts, sometimes I missed the targets even though I swam all out.

My attitude in those situations wasn't the best. In the pool, when I looked at my sports watch and discovered I had missed the target, I blurted out loudly, "Shoot!" Other times, I shocked myself by punching the water. When the rest intervals were longer, I sometimes laid my head on the deck and cried after missing a target. During bike intervals on country roads when no one was around, I sometimes yelled in frustration after I missed a target. No words came out, just a frustrated "Ahhhhh!" Sometimes I yelled so loudly into the corn-fields that I developed a sore throat. After a missed run interval, I'd put my hands on my knees and sob.

It's hard to explain those tears. I didn't feel sad or sorry for myself, and I never felt discouraged. I think my tears were a result of many things—a perfect storm of emotion and exhaustion. During the intervals, I focused intensely, held myself together through pain as the lactate built in my muscles, and hoped to hit the target. Then, when I saw the missed target, my body just released all the tension and disappointment in the form of tears. Normally, that level of dis-appointment wouldn't have brought about tears, but at the end of a hard interval when I was exhausted, I didn't have the strength to deal with my emotions, so they just came out. The tears never lasted more than a few seconds. The disappointment quickly turned to resolve: "OK, you missed that one. Let's nail the next one."

Since I was Coach Brant's eyes and ears when he wasn't at my workouts, I always reported my tears. In my narrative, I'd write, "I cried today." Coach Brant was not OK with my tears. He told me that elite athletes don't cry. They don't have lows, and they don't have highs. They keep their emotions on an even keel. He explained that some days will just be off days, and I needed to understand and accept that. I remembered Mark Allen's comments about fallback goals and changed my approach. On the days when I couldn't hit the targets, I started asking myself, "OK, what *can* you hit today?" Then I'd make that my fallback target. I also learned that while hitting targets was fun, it was not the purpose of the workout. Workouts were designed to tax my body, and even if I missed a target slightly, my max effort still achieved the impact we wanted to have. Slowly, I stopped crying in workouts.

I'd like to report that I relished each day of training, but that wasn't always the case. On some days, I dreaded working out. I just didn't have the motivation to go to the pool, run, or ride my bike. I always shared these feelings with Coach Brant to help him decide if my lack of motivation, or "mojo" as we called it, was due to fatigue. If so, he would give me a lighter workout or extra rest day. But most of the time, we decided that my lack of motivation was just one of those things.

No elite athlete, even an Olympian, wants to train every day. My hero Gwen talked about motivation as something we can't control; she said you can't always control your motivation, but you can control your discipline. So on the days I didn't feel like training, I trained anyway. I put a sign in my locker at the pool to remind me what to do on low-mojo days. It says, "Clock in. Do your absolute best. Clock out."

Beyond all of my strength, endurance, and interval training, I focused on free speed. Free speed is speed you can gain without expending energy. I told Coach Brant that if I could find ten places where I could save six seconds, I'd be a whole minute faster. Some of my free speed wasn't exactly free. I purchased a new bike. This one was also a Cervélo, but unlike my other bike, my new Cervélo P3 was designed specifically for triathlon, with two sets of handlebars. One set, the pursuit bars, were like normal bike handlebars, but the other set were aerobars. Basically, the aerobars jut out in front of the bike with armrests at the base to hold your elbows. The aerobars allow you to hold your torso parallel to the ground with your arms and hands out in front of you. This position makes you faster by cutting down on air resistance.

I also added special wheels with eight-inch rims that would help with aerodynamics. I loved the name of their manufacturer: Zipp. Finally, I purchased bike shoes and pedals that would allow me to clip my bike shoes into the pedal. This setup attaches my body to my bike, allowing my legs to work more efficiently and resulting in more power on the pedals. With all of that, my bike cost more than my first car. My husband and I were not rich, but with our house paid off, our sons through college, and income still coming in from our jobs, we were able to purchase my dream bike.

After I acquired the bike, my next step was to meet with Dave Ripley, a highly respected bike fitter, who would adjust my bike's pedals, seat height, and handlebar position so I could get the most power out of my legs, be the most aerodynamic, and have the greatest comfort. Still overweight, I worried that my belly would hit the bike's frame when I bent over to put my elbows in the aerobar's armrests. Rip had me sit on a special machine that had a seat, pedals, and aerobars. Then he told me to pedal as the machine changed the position of the seat, pedals, and aerobars. When he was finished, Rip said, "You are strong. I'm going to give you an aggressive fit."

No one had ever called me strong before, and my confidence swelled. An aggressive fit would put me in a position where my torso was more horizontal, almost like lying down on the bike. Rip added, "Don't let anyone tell you that you can't handle this fit. You are strong. You can handle it." Rip saw something in me that I didn't see in myself, and I often repeated his words as a mantra during the bike portion of races later that year: *You are strong. You are strong. You are strong.*

On the way home from my bike fit, I stopped at a trail for my first ride on my new bike. The weather was nice, but the wind was a steady thirty miles per hour with gusts. As I started to ride, I could hear the wind howling through the trees, and then *bam!* The wind hit the wide rims of my Zipp wheels and knocked me sideways. As I heard more gusts coming, I braced for each and began talking to my bike. "OK, Bike. Here comes a gust. We can do this." *Bam!* Noting that we were still upright, I continued talking. "Nice job, Bike! We did it!" Without realizing it, I had given my bike the name Bike. Not too original, but I liked it.

In addition to finding speed in my equipment, I also looked for free speed in transition from swim to bike to run. I analyzed every part of my transition. How could I get out of my wet suit faster? How could I get on my bike faster? How could I put on my running shoes faster? I found I could save time by doing two things at once. For example, as I pulled my right foot out of my wet suit, I also put on my bike helmet. I learned how to get off my bike when it was still rolling, and I stopped wearing socks during the bike and run, so I wouldn't have to spend time putting them on.

I practiced transition in front of my house. Wearing my tri kit, wet suit, swim cap, and goggles, I stood in the road and pretended it was a lake. Making swimming motions with my arms, I'd "swim" to the pretend beach at the foot of my driveway and then run up the drive to my bike, which waited at the top of the drive. As I ran, I took off my swim cap and goggles, and I peeled off the top half of my wet suit. When I reached my bike in the pretend transition area, I kicked off the bottom half of my wet suit with my feet, as my hands put on my glasses and helmet. Then I ran down the driveway, pushing my bike ahead of me, and mounted when I got to the road (which was now the bike course). After one loop around the cul-de-sac on my bike, I'd come back to transition, jump off my bike, and run around the cul-de-sac. When I completed the run, I'd put on all my tri gear and do it all again. Our neighbors came out to see what was going on. I'm sure they had a good laugh.

Finally, we looked for free speed in my technique. Sometimes just holding your body a different way can make a big difference in speed. Coach Brant started meeting with me weekly to work on technique. My biggest need for improvement was in the run. Because I was a heavy person for so many years, my natural run form was standing totally upright as my feet took fast but tiny steps. While most people struggle to get to the desired 180 steps per minute, my rpms were at 208. I looked like one of those cartoon animals whose bodies move across the screen with no vertical oscillation as their little legs move back and forth quickly. Coach Brant warned that I needed to be patient with my run. He explained that parts of my body would need to get stronger before my form could change.

All fall, winter, and spring, we turned over every stone we could find and earned speed from training, strength building, nutrition, and recovery. Coach Brant said we were putting money in the bank and that we'd make a withdrawal at Nationals. We did our best to find all of the available free speed through changes in my technique, equipment, and transition strategies. The final stone was my weight. Every pound lost would make me faster in the run, and I continued to watch my weight decrease as my strength and fitness grew.

Chapter 10

WHO AM I?

E ach morning, I stood on the bathroom scale before putting on my clothes. It was a routine: wake up; make my bed; stand on the scale; get dressed. If I had detoured from my nutrition plan for some reason, I dreaded seeing the number. But if I had stayed on plan for days, I waited in eager anticipation with the hope of seeing a lower number than the day before.

The numbers didn't always make sense. Sometimes after I'd follow my nutrition plan perfectly, I'd gain three pounds for no apparent reason. But when I thought about it, I could usually find an explanation. I might have eaten something salty or weighed myself earlier in the morning. I'd tell myself to be patient. Usually, unexpected gains were followed by unexpected losses, and vice versa. But normally, when I stayed on plan, I lost a steady two pounds a week, month after month.

I celebrated the milestones as they passed. It was thrilling to see my weight dip below 300 pounds for the first time, then 275 and 250. Strangely, no one seemed to notice that I was losing weight for the first 85 pounds. No one said anything.

When I reached 250, my old clothes began falling off me—literally. If I wasn't careful, my pants would simply slide to the ground. The only fashions available in size 5X, my size before I began losing weight, were big, blousy, and baggy. But now, at size 24, I could find fitted clothes that accented my shrinking waistline.

I found a clothing chain called Dress Barn that carried nice brands in size 24. It was wonderful to be able try on clothes in a store instead of buying 5X clothes online and hoping they would fit when they arrived. On my first shopping spree at Dress Barn, I purchased half a wardrobe. When I checked out, the owner asked if I would consider modeling for an upcoming event they were holding. Being asked to model filled me with confidence.

When I started wearing my new size 24 clothes, people finally started noticing that I was losing weight. I think my old tent-like outfits had just made it impossible to see my shrinking size. I loved when people asked me if I had lost weight, and I would happily tell them how much weight I had lost: "72.3 pounds as of this morning!" But many people were hesitant about saying anything. I suspect they were following a norm common in the United States that it's impolite to comment about another person's body. Instead they'd say, "You look fantastic! Do you have a new hairstyle?" That opened the door for me to volunteer that I had lost weight—which I always did.

During past diets, I never told people I was on a diet or how much weight I'd lost. But this time was different. This time, there was something unbelievable about my weight loss, even to me. I found myself wanting to tell everyone, "This amazing thing is happening to me."

One man really tickled me. I saw him frequently at workshops where I served as the presenter. At one workshop, he came up and whispered in my ear, "May I ask you something personal?" I wasn't sure what he was going to ask. He continued, "Have you lost weight?" After that, my weight loss seemed like a personal secret we shared. Every time he saw me, he'd whisper, "You look great!" His kindness always filled my heart.

After I lost 100 pounds, I got a different reaction when I told people how much I had lost. After I said, "I've lost 119 pounds," they'd start to say politely, "Oh, that's great." But then they'd stop in midsentence and say, "Wait. Did you say *one hundred* and nineteen pounds?" I learned to say slowly, "One hundred [*pause*] and nineteen pounds."

People always had two questions when they found out how much weight I had lost. How did you do it? And do you feel better? I always explained that I had just started eating a healthy diet and exercising, and yes, I felt great. It's wonderful to be able to tie my shoes and fit into restaurant booths. But sometimes I'd get a third question: Do you have excess skin? At first, this question left me at a loss. It seemed so personal. I wondered what they would say if I asked about one of their body parts. "Excuse me, do you have a big butt?" The questions about my excess skin seemed so invasive, so insensitive. Then I realized that they were just curious and didn't mind answering their question.

I do have excess skin. But here's the thing. Skin is really, really thin. Pinch the skin on the back of your hand. That's the thickness of skin. When I had what appeared to be big bulges of skin, it was really skin over bulges of fat. I still had weight to lose. When I lost that weight, the bulges gave way. Also, I lost the weight slowly and exercised, which gave my skin time to shrink. And finally, I discovered the miracle of spandex.

One downside of my weight loss and excess skin was that the change in my body composition affected my swim performance. While my speed in the bike and run had been increasing, I was getting slower in the swim. At first, Coach Brant and I were puzzled, but then a light bulb went off. I wondered if having less fat mass was making me slower in the swim. Fat is less dense than water, so it floats on top of the water. When I was a heavier person with a lot of fat composition in my thighs, my legs naturally rose to the top of the water. That gave me a more streamlined position, making it possible to swim faster. As I lost the fat in my legs, they sank and started dragging through the water, making me slower. To compensate, I started working on swim techniques that would help keep my sinking legs on top of the water.

I wondered if the excess skin in my legs also created drag in the water. As an experiment, I wore triathlon shorts during a swim workout to compress the skin in my thighs. Shockingly, my time per hundred meters decreased by twenty seconds! In the world of swimming, cutting twenty seconds from a hundred-meter swim is huge. Today I never swim without tri shorts over my bathing suit to make my body more streamline in the water. In races, I wear a wet suit or swimskin that compresses me from shoulders to knees. When I wear those, I feel like I'm flying through the water—and I am.

My favorite perspective on excess skin came from my eldest granddaughter. All grandmothers think their young grandchildren are the smartest, most beautiful little kids in the entire world, and I am no exception. At age four, Harper began to demonstrate her capacity for kindness and compassion. When my husband and I visited her preschool for Grandparent's Day, we were touched when she noticed a little boy playing by himself and asked him to join her play group. Another day, Harper and I were sitting on the couch, watching TV, when she started gently rubbing my upper arm. "Grandma, your skin is so soft," she said absentmindedly. Wanting to reinforce her kindness, I replied, "Harper, you always have something kind to say to people. That's a nice thing. You make people feel good." Harper didn't miss a beat. She looked up at me with her big brown eyes and said very sincerely, "Grandma, I *love* your flappy arms." Out of the mouths of babes! Harper taught me that attractiveness is based on one's perspective, and I highly valued the perspective of my sweet granddaughter.

• • •

As I prepared for my third triathlon season, when I hoped to qualify for Team USA, I continued to lose 2 pounds per week and began approaching another milestone: 164 pounds. According to the U.S. Centers for Disease Control's Adult BMI Calculator, someone my height (five feet, eight inches) would have a "normal" weight status at 164 pounds. In other words, I would no longer be considered overweight at 164 pounds. Every morning, I stepped on the scale with anticipation and watched as the number decreased: 168 . . . 167 . . . 166 . . . 165.

Then one morning, it happened. The scale read 163.9. I was no longer overweight. My reaction surprised me. I had imagined myself jumping for joy and running to post "Woohoo!" on my Facebook page. Instead, I found myself introspective and humbled. I thought about all the people who had helped me along the way: my husband and sons, Coach Brant, the folks at Meltdown Bootcamp, and all the perfect strangers who had taken time to encourage me. I shook my head and wondered how I could have lost 170 pounds. I felt so grateful that God had showered me with so many blessings.

I stepped off the scale and then stood in front of the mirror and looked at myself. Again, I felt the deep satisfaction that comes with accomplishing a hard task. At the same time, I felt unsettled. At 164 pounds, I didn't look any different than I had looked the day before at 165 pounds, but something seemed so strange. For over forty years, I had been overweight. That was my identity. But the person in the mirror was not overweight. I didn't know who she was.

My unsettled feeling continued for several weeks as I floundered with my identity. Intellectually, I knew I was no longer an obese person, but I still felt like an obese person. I had been an obese person for decades. That's who I was. My sense of self was a step behind my body. I was lost.

Coach Brant was a big help. He reminded me that I was an athlete and suggested that as my new identity. But I still struggled with thinking of myself as an athlete. I looked up *athlete* in the dictionary. Merriam-Webster defines an athlete as "a person who is trained or skilled in exercises, sports, or games requiring physical strength, agility, or stamina." I didn't feel skilled, but thanks to Coach Brant, I was certainly trained. I started practicing a little self-talk: *I am an athlete. I am an athlete. I am an athlete.* Little by little, the word seemed to feel less strange, and a new identity started to emerge. I was a mom, grandma, wife, friend, coworker, and an athlete.

When I was no longer overweight, I began thinking about the point when I would stop trying to lose weight. Although I had spent almost all my life trying to lose weight, I had never really thought about how much I wanted to weigh. I also had no experience with trying to sustain a weight, and I worried that once I stopped losing, I'd return to my old ways and go back to 335 pounds. I was afraid to stop losing weight, but I knew I had to at some point.

Around that time, Coach Brant stepped in to have a serious talk with me. He told me weight loss could be a slippery slope, and that some endurance athletes go too far and end up being so underweight that their health suffers. He wanted me to start eating more. I knew his concern came from a place of caring, and I was touched, but I did not share his concern. Throughout my journey, I had been cautious about losing weight at a reasonable pace. I had no doubt that when it came time to stop losing weight, I would do so wisely.

But where to stop? That was the big question. Every pound I took off would make it easier to run. But if I weighed too little, I could jeopardize my strength and my health. I needed to find my ideal race weight, the point where I weighed as little as possible but still had the strength I needed to push hard during training and in races.

Coach Brant wanted me to stop at 150 pounds. I respected his opinion but also sought other viewpoints. My doctor said no less than 135 pounds, explaining that I needed to weigh that much to ensure my body could take in the nutrients it needed each day. I promised my doctor that I would not go below 135. A formula based on body composition presented by a noted triathlon author indicated that I should weigh 145. But I wondered if that formula applied to me, because my excess skin affected my body composition percentages.

Finally, I found a book called *Racing Weight: How to Get Lean for Peak Performance* by Matt Fitzgerald, who had written numerous books on nutrition for endurance athletes. According Matt's formula, my ideal race weight should be between 139 and 153. I sent an email to the address on Matt's website and asked how my excess skin would affect his formula. I was surprised to receive a quick response. Matt said my question had never come up before, and he wasn't sure.

Fair enough. Not many people who have excess skin are also endurance athletes. Then he gave me some great advice. He explained that while formulas give people a general idea about the upper and lower ends of their ideal weight range, each person's ideal weight is highly individualized. He advised me to continue losing weight until I reached 153 and then to eat a little more to slow down the rate of my weight loss while paying attention to how I performed and felt. If my performance began to slide or I started to feel bad, it would be a clue that I needed to weigh a little more.

Matt's plan sounded smart to me, and when I reached 153 pounds, I started eating an extra hundred calories each day to slow my weight loss. At the same time, I wanted to be prepared to sustain my ideal weight when I got there. This is the point where I had always blown it in the past. I'd stop a diet, go back to my old eating habits, and gain it all back. I was terrified this would be one more yo-yo and that instead of sustaining my ideal weight, I'd go back to 335 pounds. I decided to seek the advice of a professional. I set an appointment with a sports performance dietitian at Indiana University, just a few miles away from my home.

I first met Brittney Bearden in the lobby of the IU football stadium. I had never been to the stadium before. As Brittney took me past the key-accessed elevator to her office, I was impressed with the facility and more than a little intimidated. Young Division I collegiate athletes passed us in the hall. They were supported by the facility's weight room, meeting rooms, and even separate dining areas, where special food to support their nutritional needs was served at all hours. I couldn't imagine professional athletes having more elaborate facilities than these college kids. As I walked down the red-and-white hallways in my spandex capris and tank top, I felt like an imposter. Once again, I reminded myself, *Go away, pride.*

Brittney started by putting me in a Bod Pod machine that would calculate my body's fat percentage. The machine looked like a cross between an egg and a space capsule with one little window. Inside was a bench, where I sat as still as possible in my bathing suit with my hair tucked under a special cap. When Brittney shut the door, the machine started making a pumping sound as it adjusted the air pressure, followed by odd clicking and clacking sounds. There was no handle inside, and I wondered what would happen if Brittney suddenly passed out. *How long would it take someone to find me? Would there be enough air to support me that long?* I quickly put those thoughts into the Do Not Think about These Things box.

When the test was over, Brittney and I sat down to talk. She told me that my body was composed of 28 percent fat, which was within the normal range. Prior to our meeting, I had sent Brittney a list of foods I ate every day, and she began sharing her concerns about my nutrition. She wanted me to eat a *lot* more calories—2,100, to be exact. I told her no way! That was more than twice the 1,000 calories I had been eating on my weight loss plan. I thought about every other time I had stopped dieting. At 2,100 calories, I knew I would regain each of the 182 pounds I had lost. I did not want to eat 2,100 calories.

Brittney had previously worked with people who were afraid of gaining weight. She seemed to understand. She didn't push. Instead, she said, "Let's just work up to 2,100 calories," and we started negotiating. She asked if I could increase to 1,400 calories. Even that sounded like a huge jump from the 1,000 calories I had been eating. Reluctantly, I agreed but added, "If I gain one pound, the deal's off."

Our plan called for me to start with 1,400 calories, and each week, we'd increase my calories a little until I was eating 2,100 per day. If I started gaining weight, we'd back off. I really didn't like the deal, but I had no alternative. I had to stop losing weight at some point, and I understood that my past plans had resulted in yo-yo diets. I put myself in Brittney's hands and hoped for the best.

Now that we had agreed on how much to eat, we started talking about what to eat. Brittney began by asking what I liked to eat. Then she created three nutrition plans that included the healthy foods that I enjoyed. I would choose a plan each day based on the duration and intensity of my workouts for that day. Each plan included breakfast, pre-workout nutrition, post-workout nutrition, dinner, and a bedtime snack. On high-intensity training days, I ate more. Her plan also increased the amount of carbohydrates and fats I ate. But the item she stressed the most was water. She encouraged me to switch all my fluid intake to plain water.

The meal plan I received from Brittney was easy to follow, since I liked the foods and had prepared them all before. I use the term *prepare* lightly. I am a not a cook, but I'm not too bad at assembling a meal by opening packages and tossing the ingredients together. And since I don't mind eating the same thing every day, meal prep was easy.

The 1,400-calorie plan I started with included the following foods. As we increased my calories, I just ate more of these foods:

51% carbohydrates (181 grams)
16% fat (24 grams)
33% protein (118 grams)

Breakfast (342 calories)
Oatmeal, 1 cup
Plain yogurt with sweetener, 1 cup
Whole-grain bread, 1 slice
Almond butter, ½ tablespoon
Multivitamin

Lunch (390 calories)
Apple, 1 large
Plain yogurt with sweetener, 1 cup
Almonds, 15
V8 juice, 11 ounces

Pre-Workout (100 calories)
Gel, 100 calories

Post-Workout (203 calories)
Protein shake, 11 ounces
Coconut water with no added sugar, 11 ounces

Dinner (266 calories)
Eggbeater egg whites, 1 cup
Spinach, 2 cups
Whole wheat bread, 1 slice

Bedtime (90 calories)
Cottage cheese, ½ cup

The plan also included a weekly cheat meal where I could eat whatever I wanted. The cheat meals had two purposes. First, they gave me a chance to eat the foods that I enjoyed on a limited basis. Second, they caused a change in the level of Leptin, the hormone responsible for suppressing hunger, making me less likely to overeat (although some debate this theory). I always used my cheat meal to eat steak and a waffle with syrup.

Brittney explained that I was still on a diet, but rather than a weight loss nutrition plan, I was transitioning to a sports performance nutrition plan. I liked the sound of that. I began thinking of food as the fuel I needed to support my training, rather than something enjoyable that I did for entertainment or to stay awake. I also found comfort in knowing that I still had a plan and that if I followed the plan, I was not likely to regain the weight as I had in the past.

I was certain that I'd gain weight on the 1,400-calorie plan, but to my surprise, I continued to lose weight, just more slowly. As I approached the start of my third triathlon season, I weighed 150 and felt great. I was ready to race and looked forward to the local races, where we would experiment with pacing strategies and I would learn how to race. And after that . . . I would compete at the USA Triathlon National Championship, attempting to qualify for Team USA.

Chapter 11

TEAM USA

I couldn't wait to begin racing in late April of my third triathlon season after seven months of preparation following season two. As planned, we started the season by using local races to test pacing strategies and help me develop the skill of racing and confidence. The USA Triathlon National Championship, where I would attempt to qualify for Team USA, was just three months away and would once again be held in Milwaukee.

Early in the season, Coach Brant experimented with my race plan to see if different paces on the bike would allow me to run faster. Slowing down on the bike portion was mentally challenging. The bike was becoming my strongest event, and I just wanted to go, go, go. But I followed Coach Brant's pacing instructions. We also experimented with pacing on the run and found a plan that worked well for me.

Coach Brant encouraged me to learn how to read my body during the run. Until that point, I had been depending on my heart rate monitor to tell me when to speed up or slow down. But during workouts and the early-season races, Coach Brant told me to judge my effort by little changes in my breathing and a funny feeling I got in my arms when I was just under the heart rate we wanted during a race.

A few weeks before one of my local races, Coach Brant told me I had to "want it" when I raced. He wanted me to be so hungry for speed that I was willing to suffer pain. I was crushed. I couldn't imagine why he thought I didn't want it enough to push through pain. After some thought about telling him how much I pushed through pain, I decided it would mean more to let my actions speak for me. Sooner or later, I figured he'd see how badly I wanted it and how much I was willing to push through pain during a race.

Pain was inevitable during hard run intervals or a race. At first, I thought every pain was an emergency, but then my sports doctor taught me how to evaluate pain. I learned to assess quickly whether the pain was from an injury and, if so, whether continuing to run would make it worse. If the answer to either of those questions was no, I'd ignore the pain, focus on my cadence, and command my body, "Do *not* slow down." Sometimes I'd trick myself into forgetting the pain by pretending to be a sports announcer: *And there's Sue Reynolds! She looks fresh! Look at her form! She's in good shape.* Sometimes I used a four-beat mantra in rhythm with my steps: *Show . . . what . . . you are . . . made of.* One of my favorite mantras was one that my brother taught me: *Looking . . . good. . . . More of . . . the same.*

My most successful strategy for dealing with the pain was to think about the science behind my effort. I knew that scientifically, I could swim, bike, and run just under lactate threshold for the entire race. I also knew that if I went over lactate threshold for more than six minutes, I'd be in trouble. My muscles would lose their ability to function.

Lactate is formed when your body breaks down glycogen for fuel during exercise. At a certain intensity of exercise, its production increases exponentially. That is lactate threshold. Coach Brant gave me swim, bike, and run tests so he could calculate my heart rate and power output at the point of my lactate threshold. In my race plans, he told me to compete at a point that was just below lactate threshold until the last six minutes of the race. Then I could push above lactate threshold, as long as I didn't push too soon.

So when the pain was intense, and my body screamed at me to stop, I would check my heart rate and power output, and if it was below lactate threshold, I'd say, Sorry body. Science says you can do this, and keep going. In the last six minutes of the race, I totally ignored my body and pushed as hard as I could. The challenge of competing at an intensity level just below lactate threshold is one of the things I enjoy about sprint triathlon.

In one of my races, I pushed too soon and scared my husband to death. I was above lactate threshold for too long, and my body started failing. I staggered down the finish chute, weaving from side to side like a drunken sailor. Two medics saw me coming and stood at the finish line, ready to assist. I felt so grateful for their support as they put my arms around their necks and carried me to the medical tent with my head flopping down to one side. Once inside the tent, they laid me on a cot, covered me with towels soaked in ice water, and gave me water to drink. I lay on the cot for a long time, enjoying the ice-cold cloths, oblivious to the race.

After that race, my husband insisted that I show the video of my staggering finish to my sports doctor. After seeing the video and asking me all sorts of questions, the doctor said, "Tell your husband my diagnosis is that you were simply exhausted." He added that exhaustion is common at endurance events.

I also shared the video with Coach Brant. I hoped seeing me stagger down the finish chute would help him understand how much I wanted it and how much I was capable of racing through pain. After seeing the video, Coach Brant never again mentioned my wanting it. I felt that Coach Brant understood what I brought to the table, and once again, the trust between us deepened.

In the end of July, we started the peak phase that Coach Brant had planned. Workouts became short and very hard. We were topping off the tank of fitness. The effort took its toll. In my exhausted state, I became cranky at home. I tried to keep from being irritable, but I wasn't very successful. I apologized and explained peak training to Brian, telling him it would be over in two weeks and asking for his patience. True to form, he showed me every kindness. I married a saint.

Finally, it was taper week—little training, lots of rest. Coach Brant told me it was time for my body to soak up all the good work we had done throughout the year. In the middle of taper week, we left for Nationals. At the time, my weight was 140 pounds. Brittney's plan was working. I continued to increase my calories each week and the pounds continued to come off, just more and more slowly. With each lost pound, Coach Brant and I studied how I felt and looked for changes in my performance during hard workouts. So far so good. I felt fine and continued to see increases in speed.

As in the previous year, I was super pumped as we left home for Nationals. The song that I sang on the way to my first Nationals popped into my head: *I'm going to Milwaukee. I'm going to the race. To see the elite women set a record pace.* I didn't think of myself as an elite triathlete, but I knew I had trained like one. I was pleased that Coach Brant and I had turned over every stone. I was curious to see what the outcome of all our work would be. We hoped for eighth place, so I could earn a position on Team USA and race at the Age Group Triathlon World Championship on behalf of the United States.

Coach Brant gave me a carefully developed race plan. I would race my heart out as I executed it. We would see what happened. As Coach Brant liked to say, "The hay is in the barn." Now we just had to race.

The race couldn't have gone better. I swam in Lake Michigan and then rode my bike and ran along the Lake Michigan shoreline. I executed Coach Brant's race plan perfectly and pushed the last six minutes per plan. That last push was painful, and I prayed for the strength to make it to the finish line. Using every mental tool possible to keep my focus off the pain, I imagined angels sweeping me off my feet and carrying me to the finish line. That didn't happen, but I did find the strength to make it to the finish—just barely. Two steps before the line, my left leg buckled. Luckily, my right leg caught my fall, and I made it across the line.

I must have looked terrible, because two men immediately told me I was going to the medical tent. There was no discussion. I remember my arms being around their necks as they led me to the tent, but I don't remember walking to the tent. I do remember the most amazing fan inside that tent. It blew ice mist, and the men positioned me in front of it. Then one opened my shirt and held out a bucket of ice. He told me to put ice in my bra. I remember thinking I should be embarrassed, but I was too out of it to care. After a while, I recovered and left to find Brian.

Brian filmed me as I walked toward him, smiling and holding my finisher medal in my hand. We found a quiet place and sat down. Immediately, I looked on my phone to see if the race results were posted. Not yet. My emotions were sky-high and full of joy. We had done it. We had worked hard all year long and left no stone unturned. We had paid attention to every little detail, turned over every stone, and lived by the motto "No excuses, whatever it takes." We had found a way around or through every obstacle. I could not have been more pleased. I remembered Gwen Jorgensen's words "I believe in process-driven goals, but I still aspire for a golden outcome." We had met all of our process goals. Now I hoped for our golden outcome—to be among the top eight finishers so I would qualify for Team USA and be able to race at Worlds.

I refreshed the results screen on my phone over and over again. Finally, the results popped up. I was eleventh.

Eleventh. Somehow, time froze, and that number just stood in front of me without any emotion attached. Eleventh. I had not made Team USA. Eleventh.

I immediately sent Coach Brant a text with just one word, "Eleventh." I knew he would be disappointed and I was disappointed too. But surprisingly, my emotions quickly turned positive. I was eleventh! I had gone from twenty-ninth to eleventh in one year! That was amazing. I was almost in the top ten, and I set a personal record in all three events. I was on top of the world and once again felt the deep satisfaction that comes with knowing I had done my best.

In a few seconds, Coach Brant sent a return text. He said he knew my finish was bittersweet, and I had done a great job. The word bittersweet jumped out at me. I knew it conveyed Coach Brant's disappointment, and that broke my heart. But it made sense for Coach Brant to feel disappointed. Just like me, he had worked hard and had high hopes. We were a team. We would celebrate together, and at times, we would be disappointed together. That's the nature of racing.

When I returned home, I thought more about placing eleventh at Nationals. If USA Triathlon hadn't changed the qualification criteria in midseason, my eleventh-place finish at Nationals would have easily put me in the top eighteen and given me a position on Team USA. In moments of self-doubt in the past year, I had sometimes doubted whether I was good enough to be on Team USA. But my eleventh-place finish at Nationals told me I was good enough to be part of the team.

With that in mind, Coach Brant and I began preparing for the second opportunity to qualify for Team USA: the new USA Triathlon Draft-Legal World Qualifier in Florida, where ten additional people would qualify for Team USA. As the race name conveyed, the World Qualifier race would be draft-legal, similar to the new race format for the Age Group Triathlon World Championship. I had two months to learn how to race in the more dangerous, draft-legal bike format.

Racing in a pack of bikes just inches from other bikes would be a new experience that required different race strategies and different skills. I needed to understand those strategies and learn those skills, so I could benefit from the lead rider in the pack, who would push the air out of my way and make it possible for me to ride faster. I also needed to overcome my fear of crashing with so many bikes close together. We needed to do a lot of work before I'd be ready for a draft-legal race.

Coach Brant started riding his bike with me during workouts. He'd simulate different situations that might occur during the race. At first, I practiced riding with my front wheel four inches behind his back wheel and a little bit to the side. I stayed slightly to the side so if he braked, my wheel wouldn't hit his. He told me to pick the side where I'd have an escape in case of a crash. If a curb was on our right, I put my wheel slightly to the left of his wheel.

Next, he taught me what to do if someone in front of me suddenly tried to surge ahead. To practice, he'd suddenly take off on his bike, and I'd quickly stand on the pedals, hit the gas, and go with him. I felt as if we were little kids playing cat and mouse, and I loved the challenge. Then, to build my confidence, Coach Brant rode next to me and bumped my shoulder or shoved my hand. I quickly learned that I could withstand a lot of bumping without going down. Finally, he invited other triathletes in the area to join us for a couple of bike workouts, so I could get comfortable in a pack of bikes.

When Brian and I left for Florida, I felt confident and ready. Coach Brant would join us a few days before the race, so he could coach me in person.

On race day, the Florida weather was unbearably hot and humid. I set up my bike and run gear in transition and then went to the swim start to do a quick warm-up swim. But when I got there, I learned they had closed swim warm-up early, and I couldn't get in the water. I knew I should put that unexpected change in the box labeled Chaos, but my emotions got the best of me, and I promptly started a pre-race meltdown. "My hair's not even wet!" I sobbed. Coach Brant instructed me to take off my swim cap, and then he poured his bottle of water over my head. That did the trick. I was ready.

This race included yet another kind of swim start I hadn't experienced before. We lined up behind a rope that lay across the Lake Louisa beach. When the horn blasted, we ran down the beach and into the lake. Per our plan, I ran into the water until it was just above my knees and then dove forward into the water, pushed off the bottom, and dove forward again. I kept dolphin diving until the water was so deep that I couldn't push myself into the air anymore, and then I started swimming.

In contrast to the blazing-hot day, the cool water felt wonderful during the swim. A swimmer who was just a little faster than I swam past me, and I was able to get behind her to draft as she pushed the water to the side for both of us. When we reached the swim exit, I ran excitedly from the water to transition over burning-hot blacktop and begin my first draft-legal bike leg.

The bike course was four laps around a three-mile loop, twelve miles in total. I had to make sure I rode four laps, not three or five. On the first lap, I rode by myself and screamed "One!" as I finished the lap. On the second lap, a group of eight younger women rode past me. As Coach Brant had taught me, I immediately stood, turned on the gas, and caught them. I was now in a pack—and I loved it.

One of the women took charge and said things like, "Let's be safe, ladies." Most of the women took turns being in front of the pack to push the air to the side as the group moved along. After each woman took her turn in front, the woman in charge yelled, "Nice job!" It was incredible to see how everyone worked together. When we looped around the start, I could hear Coach Brant cheering for me as I sped past: "Good job, Sue. Right there, Sue. Stay right there! Good work!" I could tell from his voice that he was both excited and pleased to see me holding my own in the pack of bikes. I was overwhelmed with happiness.

The run was hot, hot, hot, and right from the start, my heart rate skyrocketed from the heat. I pushed hard but also needed to keep my heart rate in the safe zone until the last six minutes, so my pace was crazy slow. With six minutes to go, I started to push. As I approached the finish line, I could hear Brian and Coach Brant yelling, "Goooooo, Suuuuuue!" After I finished, I had nothing left. Once again, the volunteers came over to see if I needed medical help.

But Coach Brant sprinted to my side and told the volunteers I would be fine. Brian found ice, and we shoved it everywhere.

I told Coach Brant that I didn't think I had gone fast enough to be in the top ten. I was so slow on the hot run. This time, the results were taped to a board near transition, where a crowd of people were all trying to find their name in the results. I squeezed my way to the front, found my name, and then spontaneously screamed, "We did it!"

I was second. Second! I qualified for Team USA. I would compete on behalf of my country the following year at the Age Group Triathlon World Championship in Cozumel, Mexico. Coach Brant had taken an obese woman with no high school or collegiate athletic experience and turned her into a Worlds-qualifier. Unbelievable. I couldn't help but get a little choked up. We did it!

Later that evening, I reflected on the past year and what had driven me to attempt to qualify for Team USA and do all the work it took to get there. It wasn't ego, pride, fear, or a lack of confidence. I didn't feel anxious or uneasy when I wasn't training. I finally decided that the driving force was joy.

I loved learning, and triathlon provided so many opportunities to learn about multiple sports and how to do each sport better. I loved solving mental puzzles and enjoyed studying my data each evening as I sought insight into how I could be faster. I loved playing games and had fun inventing games like Hit-the-Target during workouts. I loved being outside and doing the things I had enjoyed so much as a kid—running, biking, and swimming. But most of all, I believe I was motivated by my crazy curiosity. I just kept wondering, What would happen if—? and then enjoyed doing what I needed to do to find out.

Also, there was the joy of going through the triathlon journey with people who brought goodness into my life. Sharing my life with Brian was a joy. His love and support were beyond anything I had ever known, and I knew I was blessed to have a husband who was willing to sacrifice so I could chase my triathlon dreams. Sharing a common athletic goal with Coach Brant brought richness to my life, and his zany sense of humor kept me laughing. The happiness I found within the triathlon community, coupled with the kindness of perfect strangers, filled me with joy. Triathlon just seemed like the happiest place on earth.

With season three coming to a close, I couldn't wait to prepare for Worlds as a team of two with Coach Brant. I looked forward to traveling to Cozumel, Mexico to race as a member of Team USA. There would be hard work, probably harder than any work I had done to that point. But once again, my driving curiosity kicked in, and I wondered what would happen at Worlds if Coach Brant and I really worked hard in the coming year—no stone unturned, no excuses, whatever it takes.

TRIATHLON SEASON 4

WORLD CHAMPIONSHIP

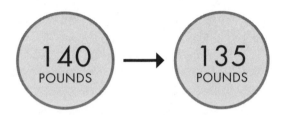

Chapter 12

BUILDING THE TEAM

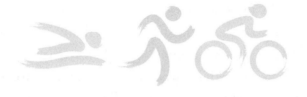

The Age Group Triathlon World Championship would be held in Cozumel, Mexico, in September at the very end of my fourth triathlon season. We had ten months to prepare for the race, and we needed it. Lots of hard work—physical and mental—lay in front of me.

One of my first tasks was to continue losing weight. At the end of season three, I weighed 140 pounds and could lose five more before hitting my doctor's 135 limit. Per Brittney's plan, I had continued to increase my calories and was eating around 1,800 calories per day. My weight loss had slowed to a crawl, but slowly the weight came off. I felt great and my performance in workouts continued to be on target. And then I hit 135 pounds. It was hard to believe that my days of losing weight were over. Once again, I felt that wonderful satisfaction that comes with completing a difficult task. I increased my calorie intake slightly and began sustaining 135 pounds, hopefully for the rest of my life.

When I looked in the mirror at 135 pounds, I saw an athlete with muscles. Seeing muscles surprised me at first. But then it made sense, given how hard Coach Brant had worked me during the previous season. I wondered if I could flex my muscles the way bodybuilders do. Feeling a little silly, I stood in front of the mirror and tried to flex a muscle. Nothing happened. But after a while, I learned that if I really focused, I could make a little muscle pop out. My new identity was taking hold. I was an athlete with strong muscles.

From time to time, I still struggled to think of myself as thin, although if I lost one more pound, I would be underweight according to my doctor. Sometimes, when I looked in the mirror, I was still surprised to find that I was not obese. All in all, though, I was happy with my progress. I loved being able to do the things I couldn't do when my body was large, like tie my shoes, fit in restaurant booths, and run and bike faster. While I've never been consumed with my appearance or the latest styles and I believe all sizes are beautiful, it was fun to try on size 8 clothes in a store after ordering size 5X online. I enjoyed wearing clothes that were more formfitting. Yes, it was tempting to be upset by my excess skin, but I chose to focus on my more positive bulges: my muscles.

Coach Brant outlined my physical training for season four. He explained that athletes aren't able to maintain a peak level of fitness over time. So he would stop assigning the short, intense intervals I had been doing at the end of the previous season. Instead, we'd go back to a base phase, where I'd do longer workouts with less intensity. Then once again, as spring and summer approached, the workouts would become shorter and harder with the aim of building a fitness level that was even greater than my fitness in season three. We planned several local races during the summer months, but this year I would have two A races. First, I'd compete again at the USA National Championship in August where, hopefully, I'd qualify for a second year on Team USA. A month later, I'd compete in my first Worlds.

Throughout the fall and winter months, the workouts were long, easy, and not very exciting. Without the intensity, my fitness slid downhill. I stopped being able to hit paces that had been easy to do. That was all part of the plan, but it was difficult to see my fitness decline. I worried that I wouldn't be able to build my fitness back to the level where it had been. But I knew I had to trust Coach Brant, and training went on day after day, week after week, month after month.

I started reading everything I could find about the Age Group Triathlon World Championship. People described Worlds as the Olympics for age-group triathletes. Each country had a system in place for selecting its best athletes to compete for medals in different age groups. Australia, Canada, Great Britain, Mexico, and the United States always sent the most athletes, but dozens of other countries also sent competitors. At the end of the week of racing, a medals count would be announced at a closing ceremony. People wrote online about how honored they were to wear their country's uniform and compete on behalf of their country.

In January, USA Triathlon began sending monthly emails to the members of Team USA. A team coach had been selected, and we started receiving suggested workouts, which I forwarded to Coach Brant. I learned there'd be a team hotel, where a team doctor, chiropractor, massage therapist, and bike mechanics would be housed during the week before the race. The more I learned, the more excited I became. My excitement shot through the sky when I received information about how to order the parade outfit, which Team USA members would wear during the Parade of Nations, and our Team USA uniform, a blue triathlon kit adorned with stars and stripes.

Training continued to go well, but the more I learned about Worlds, the more my head became a mess full of intense pressure. In the past, I had been an unknown in the triathlon community. No one had expectations of me. But now that I was part of Team USA, it felt like everyone had expectations. I wasn't under the radar anymore. I remembered how I had observed a woman at our YMCA while thinking, *She's an Ironman!* I wondered if people were now looking at me as I trained while thinking, "She's on Team USA." I wanted to tell everyone, "Yes, I'm on Team USA, but it was kind of a mistake. I'm just a beginner."

I knew USA Triathlon, as the governing body for triathlon in the United States, had invested in the team, and I worried that I'd disappoint them and all of the sponsors they had lined up for the team. Sometimes I felt as if I had to do well for every person in the entire United States of America. But most of all, I didn't want to disappoint Coach Brant. He put so much time and energy into coaching me. I wanted my performance at Worlds to please him. In addition to the pressure, there were also fears about the unknown. In many ways, I was clueless about Worlds, and I knew it.

Occasionally, I had meltdowns—periods of sheer panic when I wondered what I had gotten myself into and would burst into tears. After crying, I'd be upset with myself for being weak. Elite athletes didn't cry. But then I'd remind myself that it was reasonable for me to be scared. I was on a fast track. I had gone from not being able to tie my own shoes to qualifying for the Age Group Triathlon World Championship in a three-year period. No wonder I felt freaked out.

In the middle of meltdowns, I usually wrote to Coach Brant. He was so good at saying just the right thing to calm me down.

Sometimes Coach Brant would talk to me about God, telling me that there's nothing to fear when you have faith in God: "Nothing brings peace or a life free from anxiety other than trust in God." Other times, he would say something reassuring, like "We are going to be just fine. It's all going to work out as it should. Deep breath. All is well." It always made me feel safe when he said "we" instead of "you." The word *we* reminded me that I wasn't in this alone. Coach Brant was part of the team, too.

I started to wonder if Coach Brant would consider coming to Worlds to coach me on site before and during the race. After talking it over with Brian, I asked Coach Brant what he thought about the idea. I explained that I wouldn't be able to pay for his time, but I would cover his expenses. I hoped that the experience of going to Worlds with an athlete would make the trip worth his while. He talked over the idea with his wife and then agreed. My husband and my coach would both be there to support me at Worlds.

Throughout the fall and winter, my relationship with Coach Brant began evolving. We lived relatively close to each other, and I was able to meet his wife, daughter, and two young sons. His kids reminded me of my grandchildren, and I always looked forward to seeing them. Coach Brant also got along well with my husband. They talked about the things they had in common—working on engines, home repairs, and especially fishing.

While our conversations had always been about my triathlon dreams, we began talking about Coach Brant's triathlon dreams, too. He talked about building Dream Big Triathlon Coaching into a business that would support his family. And then one day when we met for training, he proudly announced that he had quit his job and was now a full-time triathlon coach. I loved hearing Coach Brant talk about his dreams and all the things he did to make those dreams a reality. He recruited new athletes, published articles in triathlon magazines, and began offering Dream Big triathlon clothing for his athletes to wear during races. I looked forward to cheering for my Dream Big teammates at local races in the coming summer.

At first, my changing relationship with Coach Brant confused me. He was becoming a friend, but he wasn't like any of my other friends. He was half my age, and we didn't hang out together outside of races and training. More and more, he reminded me of my own sons, and on several occasions, Coach Brant told me that I reminded him of his mother. I didn't have any category for our relationship, so I made up a new one: we were intergenerational friends.

I liked the concept of intergenerational friendship. I hoped my life experience gave me wisdom that I could share with Coach Brant, and I enjoyed his youthful zaniness, idealism, and hope. One day, when we were doing a bike workout, Coach Brant broke out in song as we rode past a sycamore tree. At the top of his lungs, he sang, "Zacchaeus was a wee little man, and a wee little man was he. He climbed up in a sycamore tree, for the Lord he wanted to see." Another time I advised Coach Brant, based on my business experience, about providing citations for quotes on his website. I began thinking the world might be a better place if we all had intergenerational friendships.

Just like all friendships, our developing relationship went through stages. During the first two years we worked together, we were in a stage with defined roles that kept us both on our politest behavior. But as we began preparing for Worlds, we started the clashing stage, when people start to be more frank and less patient with each other. Many friendships end during this phase of relationship development, and I feared that might be case for Coach Brant and me, too.

The clashes always occurred when one of us failed to meet the other's expectations. I didn't meet Coach Brant's expectations when I didn't follow his workouts as written. Once, I was supposed to swim a series of fifty-meter intervals (two lengths of the pool), with each interval lasting exactly one minute and ten seconds. But I was having a good day and wondered if I could break a minute. In my mind, that was a big milestone, and curiosity took hold as I wondered if I could do it. So, on the last interval of the workout, I ignored Coach Brant's target and sprinted as hard as I could. I finished in fifty-nine seconds—just under a minute, a new personal record. In my narrative about the workout, I told Coach Brant that I had broken a minute for the first time ever. But Coach Brant was *not* pleased. He wrote a long email to me and scolded me for swimming the last interval too fast. He asked, "What were you trying to prove?"

Another time, I felt that Coach Brant had let me down. For some reason, he failed to send feedback for a couple of my workouts. At first, my feelings were hurt. I thought Coach Brant didn't care about my training anymore. But then I thought the situation was actually a job performance issue.

In both situations, Coach Brant and I ended up sitting down to talk about the problem. I appreciated how Coach Brant always wanted to get things out in the open when one of us was upset. I think he liked that about me, too. After one of our clashes, he wrote, "I appreciate your openness with all of this. Openness brings clarity."

But at times, I wasn't so open. Sometimes, when my feelings were hurt by something Coach Brant said or did, I'd back away in defense instead of bringing it to the table. Sometimes, instead of writing my usual detailed narratives about how a workout went, I'd write a few words. One time, I wrote only, "Nothing notable." In those situations, Coach Brant could tell something was wrong, and he'd ask me about it. But other times, whatever upset me festered for days before Coach Brant noticed.

After one of those times, Coach Brant reminded me, "This is what I want from you. The moment something bothers you, I want you to tell me. There's no sense worrying about things for days and possibly losing sleep. We don't want to give molehills time to become mountains." I struggled with his message. While the trust between us had grown, I still worried that I'd hurt his feelings, or that he'd decide he didn't want to coach me anymore. But as I had done so many other times since starting my journey, I told my fear to go away, and I initiated a talk with Coach Brant about what was bothering me.

Every time I opened up about my concerns, the result was positive. Sometimes Coach Brant told me I had misinterpreted something he had said or done, and he'd explain what he was thinking at the time. Other times, Coach Brant agreed that I had a legitimate concern, and he apologized and changed his actions immediately. That response impressed me so much.

Our coach-athlete relationship and intergenerational friendship slowly moved out of the clashing stage and into a new stage marked by respect, trust, and free-flowing communication. And in this new stage, we prepared productively for Worlds.

In late winter, our trust and strong communication enabled us to work through a new hurdle. I began feeling beaten down by Coach Brant's critiques when he coached me face-to-face. At one swim workout alone, he found fault with my hands, arms, head, hips, legs, and feet. Only my hair escaped criticism (probably because it was hidden under my swim cap). I also noted that the positive feedback I used to receive on a regular basis had disappeared. I missed hearing "Well done!" or "Nailed it!" when I did a tough workout with integrity.

I told myself that I wasn't performing for Coach Brant's praise, and I tried focusing on being internally motivated. I reminded myself of all the things I loved about triathlon. I gave myself positive feedback when I did something well. But it just wasn't the same as hearing "Nice job!" from my coach. I hungered for validation to let me know I was doing something right in addition to all the things that Coach Brant was telling me that I was doing wrong. I found it difficult to keep my spirits up under the deluge of critique.

Thankfully, I could now talk to Coach Brant about the things that bothered me. I explained the situation to him and asked if he could use constructive praise in addition to constructive criticism. Coach Brant didn't agree with my observation. He felt that he had been pointing out what I did well and that I might be overly focused on his corrections. He added that he critiqued my performance because he believed in me and wanted to see me improve. Coach Brant also explained that his view of me had changed. In his mind, I was a Worlds-qualifier, a committed athlete who no longer needed lots of encouragement. Doing hard workouts with integrity was just part of the routine. But Coach Brant also heard what I was saying, and I noted that he immediately started adding constructive praise to his comments. The praise wasn't routine. I had to earn it by doing something significant. But when I did, I started hearing "Nailed it!" in his comments once again.

The summer months were quickly approaching. Coach Brant and I shared a new level of trust, and my training was going well. Over the fall, winter, and spring, we had built a strong base of fitness and were now in the build phase of training, with shorter and harder workouts. Soon we would begin my local races, where I would get race experience and Coach Brant would continue testing different pacing strategies. All was well, and then it wasn't.

Chapter 13

CATASTROPHE, FAITH, AND COZUMEL

K aren is going in for some tests. She may have cancer." Time stopped. I couldn't believe what Coach Brant had just said. Karen may have cancer. He explained that his wife had found a lump in her breast and her doctor had verified it. The tests would tell if the lump was cancer. Karen was only twenty-nine years old. She was much too young to have cancer. I was sure the test results would be negative. Still, I had experienced a similar scare several years earlier and remembered the agonizing feeling of waiting for the test results.

In the days that followed, without telling people why, Coach Brant posted Bible verses on Facebook. One post said, "'Trust in the Lord with all your heart, and do not lean on your own understanding. In all your ways acknowledge him, and he will make straight your paths' (Proverbs 3:5–6)."

The test results came back positive. Karen had cancer. She would begin chemotherapy immediately. My heart broke for Coach Brant and his family.

Three days after Coach Brant learned that his wife had cancer, he and I were scheduled to do a face-to-face bike workout. I wrote to Coach Brant, "What's the plan for tomorrow? Remember, from my perspective, it's family first. Canceling or postponing is not an issue. There's nothing that can't wait." I assumed that Coach Brant would cancel the one-on-one coaching session we had scheduled, but he did not.

When Coach Brant showed up at my house for our bike workout, all I wanted to do was give him a big hug and tell him how sorry I was. But as soon as he walked in the door, he acted as if everything was normal, as if his wife didn't have cancer, as if his world hadn't just fallen apart. I assumed we would talk for a while before getting on our bikes for a training ride, but I was wrong. He wanted to get straight to training. Looking back, I can now see that I was the one who needed to talk. Out of concern for Coach Brant and his family, I wanted to know how he and Karen were doing. I wanted to help. But that's not where he wanted to go. He wanted to train. I followed his lead, and we jumped on our bikes.

The training ride seemed strange. We worked on gearing over rolling hills. I kept wanting to say, "Brant, your wife has cancer. How can we be riding our bikes like everything is normal?" But I didn't say anything. I just tried to switch my bike gears at the right times. We acted normal.

When we got back to my house, I asked Coach Brant a few open-ended questions to create an opportunity for a conversation. Coach Brant explained that he was not upset. There was nothing to worry about. Karen was in God's hands. He explained that God is good all of the time, even when we don't understand God's ways. He explained that God doesn't always grant us our wishes but is always good. He and Karen were committed to God's will, even if it meant that Karen would leave this world.

I couldn't imagine a faith that strong, and I questioned him. "I hear you saying that God is good, but underneath, doesn't this situation concern you a little bit?" Again, Coach Brant emphasized, "God is good all the time," and he repeated that he and Karen accepted God's plan, whatever that might mean. I remembered Coach Brant telling me we should focus on heavenly things, not earthly things. I was beginning to understand that, for Coach Brant, even life itself was an earthly thing. I was completely awed by the strength of his faith.

Coach Brant had often told me that we should use our gifts to bring glory to God. He often said, "Let your light shine." Now I saw how Coach Brant was using his catastrophe to bring glory to God. On social media, when finally writing about Karen's cancer, he said, "We know the Lord is always good, and that He has us in His hands and will carry us through this." Witnessing Coach Brant's peace and his trust that God is always good spoke to me deeply. I wondered if I could have that kind of faith, too. I began asking God for something far different from the requests of my younger days—good grades or bike riding or the right marriage. I started asking for the strength of faith that I witnessed in Coach Brant and his wife.

As Karen started treatments, I wanted to help badly, but I wasn't sure what to do. Then I remembered how Coach Brant had comforted me when I experienced the atrial flutter a few years back. He kept track of my doctor's appointments and sent me an encouraging text shortly before each visit. I began sending Coach Brant a supportive text before each of Karen's doctor appointments. I hoped the support of friends would help. I knew that Coach Brant took much comfort in the Bible, so I decided to send him quotes from the Bible that might be inspiring at such a difficult time. The only problem was that I didn't know how to do that. While I had listened to scripture readings at church, I had never quoted scripture. I had no idea where to begin and was afraid I'd do something wrong and sound silly.

I owned a Bible but had no clue where it was, so I ended up doing a Google search for "breast cancer scripture." I found a few passages that I liked, but I didn't know how to cite the verses. I knew you put someone's name and a few numbers after the passage, but that was it. Again, I turned to Google: "How do you cite the Bible?" Carefully, I typed my first scripture passage with a citation and proofread it a million times. Then I sent it to Coach Brant: "'I pray that out of his glorious riches he may strengthen you with power through his Spirit in your inner being, so that Christ may dwell in your hearts through faith' (Ephesians 3:16–17)." A few days later, I sent another scripture passage, and then another.

As I searched for Bible passages to send to Coach Brant, I discovered a lot of wisdom in the Bible. I couldn't understand why I had never noticed it before. I had listened to scripture readings every Sunday at church for decades, but the readings at church seemed like a foreign language. The words I read online seemed clear and meaningful. Finally, I understood there were different translations of the Bible.

The church I attended for most of my life used the Revised Standard Version of the Bible, first published in 1946. It was a second-generation revision of the King James Bible which was published three centuries earlier in 1611. Although the writers attempted to use simple words in the Revised Standard Version, many of the words and sentence structures from the 1600s remain and were difficult for me to comprehend. In contrast, the scripture I found online came from a translation called the New International Version. It used everyday English that was easy for me to understand.

I called our older son, who at that time was studying to be a pastor, and asked him which version of the Bible was the best. He explained that scholars debate that question, but in his opinion, the best Bible version is "the one that you will read." So, I decided to leave the debate about Bible translations to the scholars and continued reading the version that made sense to me, the New International Version.

The more I searched for Bible passages to send to Coach Brant, the more and more I became engaged with scripture. The passages taught great lessons. In fact, the Bible seemed like an instruction manual for life. I started reading the Bible every morning, using an app on my phone that provided daily scripture readings. I loved starting my day with words to help me feel God's love and live a kind and thoughtful life.

• • •

Throughout the summer, my local races came and went, and finally, I was at the USA Triathlon National Championship, which was held in Omaha, Nebraska. I hoped to qualify for a second year on Team USA at this race. I executed my race plan perfectly until the run. I pushed too early and ran out of steam before the finish line. Even so, I finished tenth. I was thrilled to be in the top ten in the country but disappointed to not make the top eight. Once again, I would need to attend the USA Triathlon Draft-Legal World Qualifier race to try to remain on Team USA for a second year. That race would be after the Age Group Triathlon World Championship, so I pushed it out of my mind. I'd worry about that race after Worlds.

After Nationals, we had just a few weeks to get ready to race at Worlds. While Coach Brant had planned to travel to Cozumel, Mexico with me for the race, I suggested that he not attend Worlds and instead stay home with Karen. After discussing the situation with his wife, Coach Brant told me he would be going to Worlds. He made everything seem so normal that it was hard to remember that his wife had cancer and his world was upside down. I hoped that the time in Mexico would be good for him and that he would be able to enjoy the experience.

One of the challenges of going to Worlds was figuring out how to travel with my bike and all my triathlon gear. I purchased a special box designed for transporting bikes. I packed my suitcases with triathlon gear (helmet, shoes, bike pump, etc.), training clothes, street clothes, and food for the days prior to my race. To my relief, Mexico had fairly lenient rules for bringing food into the country. I packed freeze-dried eggs, rice in boiling bags, instant oatmeal, bread, almonds, applesauce, and banana baby food. Since my hotel room didn't have a refrigerator or microwave, I also took a pan and convection burner. When fully packed, we had seven pieces of luggage. Six of them were mine. One was Brian's.

When Brian and I left for the airport, I was a jumble of emotions. Traveling to another country to race in a world championship felt surreal. I shook my head in wonder throughout the morning. I wore one of my official team shirts that said, "TEAM USA" across the front, and I walked through the airport with my head held high, pushing my bike box in front of me. One person even stopped me to ask if I was on Team USA. With a huge smile, I responded, "Yes! I am!"

We flew from Indianapolis to Dallas and then boarded a plane for Cozumel. I was surprised to find triathletes on the plane from all over the world. Evidently, everyone flew to Dallas to make the connection to Cozumel. During the flight, I chatted with athletes from Australia, Canada, and several other countries. My excitement rose, and once again I found myself shaking my head in disbelief. This was happening. I was going to Worlds.

When the plane landed in Cozumel, we walked into customs and got in line. I could see everyone's bike boxes as workers shoved them through a door into the room, and I nervously waited for my bike to appear. However, it was nowhere in sight. I started to feel a little frantic.

Then my attention suddenly shifted. A *large* black dog was racing right at me. There was no mistake about it. He was charging at me, barking and growling, and dragging a customs official behind him. I didn't know what was happening and wondered if he would knock me down or bite me. I couldn't imagine what I had done to make that big black dog charge at me.

The customs official was not exactly friendly. In fact, he was intimidating. "Do you have food in your backpack?" he demanded in a rough voice. My brain raced through everything in my pack. I knew I was not allowed to bring fresh fruit and several other food items into Mexico. I had given the flight attendant several apples before deplaning. I wondered if I had missed one. I pictured myself in jail, missing my race. I told the official no, and he demanded "Are you sure?" His tone said, "My dog never makes a mistake. I know you have food in your pack. If it's not food, then it's illegal drugs. You are going to jail." I wondered how many grandmas in their sixties smuggle drugs into Mexico. Again, I told the official that I had no food in my pack. He put a sticker on my pack and told me to get my bike and then get in a special line to have my pack searched.

I still couldn't find my bike. There must have been a hundred bike boxes, but none of them had florescent duct tape with

"FRAGILE!!!" written across it, which I'd so carefully taped to my box back home. Maybe it didn't matter. If I went to jail, I wouldn't need my bike. Finally, I saw my bike box roll through the door—a huge relief. I rolled my bike box to the station where my pack would be examined. The official looked through everything in my pack and found no food. Then she looked again. She obviously expected to find something illegal. Finally, I had a thought. The day before, I'd had Gatorade in my now-empty water bottle. Could the dog have smelled that? Yes. That was it. The official closed my pack, and we were on our way.

After Brian and I checked into the hotel, I opened my bike box and was horrified to see the front wheel facing sideways. If I rode my bike in that condition, I'd just ride around in circles! Evidently, my florescent tape and the word *FRAGILE!!!* did not keep it from being tossed around on the plane. I could loosen the bolts to move it back in place, but I didn't have the torque wrench I needed to retighten the bolts. The bike mechanics from USA Triathlon hadn't arrived yet, and I was scheduled to do a bike workout the next day. I called several bike shops, but with all the athletes in town, no one was available. My husband was good at mechanical things, but he was unable to accurately judge the feel of the specified Newton-meters. I imagined my handlebar swiveling during a training ride and began to panic. Luckily, Coach Brant would arrive the next day. With years of bike experience, he could tighten the bolt by feel.

That evening, I checked my email and social media. Our younger son sent a photo with our grandkids all wearing T-shirts that said, "Grandma's Cheer Squad" on the front. Our older son sent supporting words. And each of my colleagues at work sent a photo of the palm of their hand with the word *Sue* written on it—much as I write the names of inspiring people on my hand before I race.

The next day, Coach Brant arrived in the late afternoon. We had rented a bike for him to ride in Mexico, and after he fixed my bike, Coach Brant and I left for a training ride along the Gulf of Mexico. The ride was beautiful, with the sun setting over the water between the island of Cozumel and mainland Mexico. Our training ride turned into an adventure when the last inch of sun disappeared over the horizon, and day suddenly turned pitch black. We rode back to the hotel in the dark as Coach Brant illuminated the patch of pavement just in front of us with the light on his iPhone.

The next day, Coach Brant joined me for an easy run. We ran down the sidewalk among the Mexican tourist shops. Two days before race day, and all was well. The last day before the race, Coach Brant and I rode to the race venue, where I would leave my bike in transition overnight. Brian took a shuttle to the venue, so he could be there, too. I was pleased with my assigned spot in transition. I had a straight run from swim-in to bike-out. Perfect. Coach Brant rode his rental bike back to the hotel while Brian and I took the shuttle. That evening all the athletes marched in a Parade of Nations behind their country's flag to an Opening Ceremony. I wanted so badly to be part of parade. I had looked forward to wearing the red, white and blue USA parade outfit provided by USA Triathlon, and waving a small American flag with my teammates. However, I worried that marching the night before my race would use valuable energy that I needed to save for race day. For the umpteenth time, I asked myself, "What would Gwen do?" The answer was obvious. I decided to skip the parade and opening ceremony. I had come to Cozumel to race. No stone unturned.

As I laid in bed that evening, I realized that all the work was done. Grateful tears streamed down my face. There was only one thing left to do: race.

When the alarm rang at 3:55 the next morning, my first thought was "Race day!" My husband takes charge of keeping me on time during race mornings, since punctuality is not one of my strong points. "Time to eat," he said. I quickly downed two slices of white bread, three tablespoons of jam, two containers of banana baby food, and twenty ounces of Gatorade. A short while later, Brian said, "Put on your race numbers." I pressed temporary tattoos with the number 1250 on each arm and each leg. "Check your gear." I quickly checked to make sure I had the items I would use in the race: swim cap and goggles; bike shoes and helmet, run shoes, race bib, and water bottle. I also checked for the bike computer that would sit between the aerobars on my bike. During the race, I would monitor data like my speed, heart rate, how fast my feet were going around, and how much power I was putting into the pedals. Finally, I checked for my run computer. I'd wear that on my wrist like a watch and monitor similar data during the run.

Finally, Brian said, "Time to go!" I gave him a quick kiss, and we walked out the door—just a few minutes late. As we left, I got a text message from Coach Brant. He was already in the lobby, waiting for us. His text said, "Are you coming?" It was comforting to know that both Brian and Coach Brant were looking out for me.

We took a shuttle bus from the hotel to the race venue and then walked to transition. When we reached transition, I freaked out. The bike dismount line was a different color. Yesterday it was red. Today it was green. I didn't know why they would change the color of the dismount line and wanted to ask Coach Brant about it, but I couldn't find him. I panicked. Where was Coach Brant?! He was just a short distance away behind a tree, but I didn't know that. I had no idea where he was.

That was my breaking point, and a total meltdown followed. All of my fears about the race suddenly came to the surface. I became acutely aware that I was a virtual beginner on a world stage. I felt overwhelmed. And now, the person who knew what to do had disappeared. I felt like a terrified three-year-old who had lost her parent in the department store. I wanted to wail into the darkness, "Coach Brant!" When Coach Brant appeared, all I could do was sob, "I couldn't find you! I didn't know where you were." He calmly assured me that he was there. We walked to the dismount line, and he acknowledged that it was different than it had been the day before.

Coach Brant reminded me that at big races, many things change with little or no warning. He told me I needed to be flexible, to go with the flow without letting anything upset me on race day. As much as I had grown in my ability to manage my fears, the changing color of the dismount line had gotten the best of me. I still had a lot of growing to do.

Brian, Coach Brant, and I walked in the darkness to the entrance to transition. Since only athletes are allowed in transition, I walked into transition alone. As I walked away from Brian and Coach Brant, I turned around and gave them a smile and a big thumbs-up. I found my bike where I had left it hanging on the bike rack. My place on the rack was marked by a sticker that had an American flag and "Sue Reynolds, United States" printed on it. I became misty-eyed. The entire experience was so surreal.

I inflated my tires and panicked a little when air began coming out of my tires as I tried to inflate them. Luckily, Coach Brant was standing on the other side of the chain-link fence that surrounded the transition area. I walked my bike over to him, and he gave me instructions. The tires inflated. Phew! I attached my bike shoes to the pedals, so I could save a few seconds by mounting my bike barefoot and then slipping into my shoes while my bike was rolling. Then I put my glasses inside my helmet and hung the helmet from my handlebar. I placed my run shoes and race belt under my bike and did my usual race-morning checks. Then, as I always do, I put a hand on my bike and prayed for a safe race for everyone. So far, so good.

I always loved transition in the morning darkness. I gazed at thousands of bikes from all over the world that were waiting for their owners and thought about all the hopes and dreams they represented. As I walked back to Brian and Coach Brant, I listened to people chatting in different languages. I was touched that people from countries all over the world had gathered to compete peacefully. Suddenly, it hit me: I was competing at the Age Group Triathlon World Championship. It seemed impossible, yet it was true.

Brian, Coach Brant, and I walked to the swim start as the sun rose and the air became unbearably hot and humid. We sat on the ground in the shade and waited for my wave to be called to the start line. This was it! For the umpteenth time, I shook my head in wonder. Four years ago, I was not able to tie my own shoes, and in a few minutes, I would be racing against the best triathletes in the world.

Finally, the announcer called my wave to the first of three holding corrals, first in Spanish and then in English. My wave would progress from corral to corral. After the last corral, we would go to the start line. I was excited for me but also excited for Coach Brant. He had written the training plan that had gotten us to this point. This wasn't *my* race. It was *our* race. As the women in my wave started to congregate, I gave Brian a kiss and Coach Brant a high five, and then I walked alone to the first holding corral.

Chapter 14

WORLDS!

The official dropped the rope that separated athletes in the last holding corral from the start line at the Age Group Triathlon World Championship. I ran down the long dock that jutted into the Gulf of Mexico, leading 113 of the best triathletes in the world. After jumping into the water, I did a quick warm-up and then placed one hand on the dock next to the hands of my competitors and waited for the blast of the airhorn.

This was it. I was about to race at Worlds. While my insides had been a mess of emotions earlier in the morning, I now felt strangely calm. I had a job to do. I was ready to swim the 0.5 miles, bike the 12.4 miles, and run the 3.1 miles that stood between me and the finish line. I pressed my swim goggles hard against my eyes one last time.

Swim

"Set!" the starter said through a megaphone. The shriek of the air horn pierced the air, and my body immediately responded. I did a strong breaststroke kick to get my lower body to the surface of the water as I reached forward with one arm to begin stroking. I was out in front of the women around me. For a moment, my emotions sky-rocketed into outer space. I was swimming at Worlds! But I quickly pushed my excitement aside to focus on the task at hand.

After eight strokes, I lifted my head, with my eyes just above the water, to look for the first turn buoy. Phew, I found it. After another eight strokes, I lifted my head again and found the buoy still in sight. Good, I was on course. I started playing my checklist. Head down? Check. Quick arm rotation? Check. Strong catch at the start of my stroke? Check. Hips driving forward in a dance-like rhythm as I threw each arm forward? Check. Everything seemed to be going well. I was pleased with the start of my swim.

The course took us clockwise around a long, skinny rectangle. We started in the middle of one of the long sides, and would make four right turns around buoys on our right. Once we were around the rectangle, we would turn left around the final buoy and swim to shore. Then we'd exit the Gulf of Mexico under a large inflated arch.

The water was crystal clear, and as I swam, I wondered if I'd be able to see critters. I worried about critters that were not easy to see, especially jellyfish. Prior to the race, I had read about the jellyfish in Cozumel. Thankfully, they were not the kind that killed you. If a jellyfish stung me, I knew I should just keep swimming. I tried not to think about stingrays and sharks. Coach Brant's words came back to me. I was in God's hands, and God is always good, even when we don't understand God's logic. Whatever God had in mind for me, it was the right thing. That thought gave me peace. The stingrays and sharks stopped being so scary.

When we started the race, the 113 women in my wave had been spread out along the length of the dock, but as we swam toward the first buoy, we converged to a single point. We became a madhouse with elbows and hands everywhere. All thoughts about my form disappeared. I was just trying to make my way through the bodies. But after the second buoy, we spread out again as faster swimmers charged ahead and slower swimmers fell behind.

The muscles in my arms and back engaged, and I knew I was having a strong swim. At one point, I could feel someone's fingers on my toes repeatedly as she drafted behind me. She was able to swim faster because I pushed aside the water in front of her. Feeling her fingers on my toes didn't bother me. Drafting was just part of swimming.

Suddenly, five or six huge waves appeared. I swam into them head-on and felt my body being lifted high into the air before being gently dropped back to its original position. These were not normal ocean waves. They were gigantic rolling waves. The waves felt like they were lifting my body three stories into the air—no exaggeration. It reminded me of a roller coaster and was kind of fun.

Shortly after the waves subsided, a woman passed me and appeared to be swimming slightly faster than I swam. Great! This was my chance to draft. As she passed, I swam off her left hip for a while and then positioned myself behind her. I loved swimming through the millions of tiny bubbles she made as she swam in front of me. They almost tickled. Then I touched her toes. She went ballistic—I mean, totally ballistic. Her entire body started moving every which way, and she was kicking. It wasn't a flutter kick to propel her through the water. She was kicking with bent knees and feet flat. She was kicking *at* me! I saw the bottom of her foot coming at my face like a karate kick. Instinctively, I bent my body at the hip to stop my forward movement and jerked my head back. Thankfully, her foot did not make contact. But my sudden movement stopped me in the water, and I had to build my speed again, losing time and precious energy.

My coach wanted me to be "on the edge" as I swam the 0.5 miles. That meant I needed to swim as fast as I could without swimming so fast that I couldn't maintain the effort for the entire distance. His goal was for me to exit the water with the stronger athletes, so I could draft with them during the bike. I felt I was swimming fast, but something seemed horribly wrong as I swam the 300 meters to the third buoy. The rocks beneath me were barely moving. It was taking much longer than I thought it should take. That made no sense. I began to wonder if I was having an off day but told myself to be patient and just keep going. A woman in a green triathlon suit was swimming next to me. I could see MEX across her chest and rear end as she rotated in the water with every stroke. If I was slow, at least I wasn't alone.

Ouch! I suddenly felt an intense sting on my left calf, like a wasp sting. What was that? Was that a jellyfish? *Do not panic,* I commanded myself. *You are not going to die. Don't stop.* As I swam forward without missing a stroke, I monitored my body. No problem breathing. Heart seemed OK. Pain was not getting worse. And then I laughed to myself. If you had told me three years ago that I would keep swimming after being stung by a jellyfish, I wouldn't have believed you. Back then, I probably would have gone to the hospital. It was crazy how much my life had changed. I no longer worried about all the little things that could go wrong. I had come prepared, and I knew I was in God's hands. That peace gave me freedom to do the things I loved to do, like fly in an airplane, talk about my faith, and swim in the Gulf of Mexico after being stung by a jellyfish.

I finally reached the opposite end of the long rectangle. As I approached the third buoy, everything was fine. I swam a line that would take me just to the left of the large inflated buoy, exactly where I wanted to be. A woman next to me wanted the same line, and we reached the yellow buoy at the same time. Then she just disappeared under the six-foot-wide buoy! And then suddenly, I disappeared under the buoy. On my next breath, I saw the buoy over my head, and everything looked yellow as the sun shined through it. The other woman was nowhere to be seen. I struggled to swim from underneath the buoy, while looking for the anchor line that held the buoy to the ocean floor. I knew I had to pass on the left of that line, or I would be penalized for being off course. With huge relief, I saw the line go by on my right.

As soon as I emerged from under the buoy, I heard millions of whistles blowing in quick, rapid tweets. I could tell they were trying to get someone's attention but wasn't sure what was going on. Did I do something illegal? Were they blowing their whistles at me? The next time I sighted, I glanced at one of the officials, who sat in a kayak. Was he looking at me? No. Big relief!

On my next sighting, I saw the official motioning to a woman. Evidently, all the whistles had been at her. The official was motioning for her to swim back to the buoy we had just passed. I suspected she was the one who had disappeared under the buoy. She must have swum on the wrong side of the buoy's anchor line, and they were making her go back.

I seemed to be making good progress now, and I felt strong and fast as I swam toward the last yellow buoy. On the course map, that buoy was about fifty meters from the dock where we started. I just needed to reach that buoy, make a left turn, and swim to shore. When I reached the buoy, I started to turn left. One moment, everything was fine, and the next moment as I took a breath, my face was literally six inches from the start dock. That made no sense.

I couldn't figure out how I had gotten so far off course so quickly. Embarrassed, I tried to swim to shore, but my legs were suddenly *under* the dock. I was kicking the dock's scaffolding and cut my foot on a sharp edge. I tried repeatedly to swim away from the dock at an angle toward shore, but every time I did, my legs were under the dock again. I saw another woman with both arms wrapped around the scaffolding, apparently holding on for dear life. Finally, I swam like crazy away from the dock and then angled toward the swim exit. Thankfully, I made it.

To get from the water to my bike in transition, I had to run about a half mile. As I ran from the water, I heard the announcer say, "Here comes Reynolds from the United States!" His Mexican pronunciation of my last name (Ray-nold) reminded me that I was in an international competition. Then he added, "All smiles. The swim is officially over. Let's get ready for the bike." That was such an odd thing to say, especially because I did not have a smile on my face. I never smile when racing. I am too focused on racing. His comment was strange, just like the odd twists and turns in the water.

A few hours after the race, I learned that a rogue ocean current had hit in the middle of our swim. Now, everything made sense. The huge waves I experienced after the second turn was the start of the rogue current. The current had made the swim to the third buoy extremely difficult. When I turned to go around the third buoy, the current hit me broadside and pushed me under the buoy. My swim to the last buoy was superfast because I was swimming with the current. And then, when I swam around the final buoy, it was on the dock (where the current had pushed it), and as I turned, the current caught me broadside and pushed me under the dock.

Spectators told me later that onlookers had been terrified as they saw the situation unfold. They witnessed women in white swim caps being smashed against the dock, with some heads disappearing underneath. A couple of men jumped in the water to pull some of the women from under the dock. Everyone speculated that the reason the announcer said I had a smile on my face was to ease the panic building in the crowd. I later talked to a few women who were unable to make *any* forward progress against the current. Boats came to rescue them. Karate kick, jellyfish sting, rogue ocean current, cut foot—what a crazy swim!

Transition 1

As I ran from the water, I heard Brian and Coach Brant cheering for me. During the half-mile run to my bike, I did a quick injury check from the jellyfish sting and scaffolding kick. No pain. Good to go. I had no trouble finding my bike. During my preparation for the race, I had replaced the black handlebar tape with neon-green tape, which made my bike stick out among the thousands of bikes waiting for their owners in transition. I quickly threw my swim cap and goggles under my bike, put on my helmet and glasses, and grabbed my bike off the rack. Then I ran in bare feet as I pushed my bike ahead of me by the saddle.

Bike

For the first time ever, the sprint race at Worlds was draft legal. After my experience in the qualifying race, I looked forward to riding in packs and drafting behind other bikes. This was my second draft-legal triathlon, but since draft-legal was a new format for Worlds, most of the women competing had no experience with draft-legal racing.

I ran out of transition, crossed the mount line, placed my left foot on top of the shoe already clipped into my pedal and pushed off. My right leg swung nicely over the saddle and my bare foot found the top of my other shoe. Phew. So far, so good.

The first part of the bike course was on pavement with the texture of cobblestone. I worried that my front wheel might get caught between the cobbles and cause me to crash, but thankfully, I was able to get through that section in one piece. Once on smooth pavement, I got up to speed, slipped my feet into my shoes, and reached down to tighten the Velcro straps. Now I could pull *up* on my feet as well as push down to pedal more efficiently.

I passed several slower women, and a few of them turned on the gas to catch my rear wheel. They began drafting behind me. My bike computer showed the power I was putting into my pedals. I monitored power along with my heart rate, speed, and distance traveled. The data helped me know if I was going too hard or too easy. If I went too hard, my legs would be toast before I started the run.

About three miles into the race, I was leading a pack of five women. Ideally, everyone would take turns being the lead bike. But that wasn't happening. I was doing all the pulling. I decided to take control. "OK, ladies!" I yelled. "Let's work together!" I moved my bike to the side, and motioned back and forth with my elbow. That was the sign to the bike behind me that I wanted to be passed. As each woman passed, I said, "Thirty-second pulls. Let's do this!" Woman began taking short "pulls" at the front, before dropping back to the last position. Bingo! We were a pace line with each bike taking a turn in front and then pulling to the side before dropping to the back of the line.

The women in our little pack were from different countries: Canada, Mexico, Great Britain, and another woman from the USA. As each woman dropped back to the end of the line, I'd try to say something encouraging. "Good job, Mexico!" "Great pull, Canada!" At one point, I got a little choked up as I thought about how amazing it was to be working with women from different countries toward a common goal. I wished that countries from all over the world could work together peacefully, the way we were. We were a team on a mission.

I noticed that when I was in front, our speed was greater, so I started to take longer pulls. I knew that would tax my legs, but I didn't want to ride as slowly as they were going. Then I noticed that one of the women wasn't pulling at all. When each of us finished our pull and dropped to the back of the line, she'd brake to make room in front of her. Then she'd say, "Go in front of me." In doing so, she was always in the back, in a great position to draft and save energy for the run. I guessed that her coach had told her to do that. But maybe she was just scared.

After one of my pulls, I challenged her, "Come on. Let's all take a pull." I slowed even more than she did and pulled in behind her. But when it was her turn to pull, she couldn't (or wouldn't) keep up the pace, and the whole group ended up slowing down. At that point, I knew we couldn't count on her to pull.

Prior to the turnaround, I decided to make a break. My hope was to go hard out of the turn and lose the weaker bikes in our group. The strongest cyclist seemed to be the woman from Great Britain. As we approached the turnaround, I whispered to her that I was going to make a break and said, "Come with me!" After the turn, I cranked up the effort. Great Britain came with me, but so did the woman who refused to pull. However, we lost Mexico. She was nowhere to be seen.

On the way back to the start, we approached an accident. An ambulance's lights were flashing, and people standing along the side of the road were motioning frantically for us to slow down. I said a quick prayer for the injured cyclist. But when I looked at the road in front of us, there was no reason to slow. The road was perfectly clear. I speculated that the spectators were overreacting. Unfortunately, I was third in the pace line, and the two women in front of me slowed to an absolute crawl. Lesson learned. I need to be in front when there's anything that might make people want to slow down, so I am in control of the pace.

The bike course hugged the Gulf of Mexico as we returned to the start. The blue water under sunny skies was beautiful, although I really didn't have time to enjoy the view.

A couple hundred meters before the dismount line, I reached down and undid the Velcro straps on my shoes. Then I slipped my feet out and pedaled with them on top of my shoes. As we approached the dismount, I planned to ride hard to the line, and at the last moment, I'd swing my right leg over the saddle, jump off my bike while it was still moving, and take off running. However, the two women in front of me slowed down to a crawl again, and I was stuck behind them. Then I saw a narrow space between the two of them. As I threw my leg over the saddle, I squeezed through that space and hit the ground running. In doing so, I crossed the dismount line ahead of them. Nice!

I didn't know it at the time, but I ended up having the fastest bike split in my age group. First in bike at the Age Group Triathlon World Championship!

Transition 2

I ran into transition and panicked. I couldn't find the spot where I needed to rack my bike. There were dozens of rows of bike racks, and each long rack had hundreds of little stickers attached to it where bikes had been placed. One of those stickers marked my place in transition. In the United States, athletes put towels on the ground to mark their spot in transition, but in this international competition, towels were not allowed.

During setup that morning, I had carefully chosen a landmark to help me find my little sticker in the racks. The landmark was an orange cone that officials had put over a root in front of my bike, so no one would trip on it. I planned to look for that cone when I came into transition. But now the cone was gone. I gazed across the field and saw rows and rows of bike racks and thousands of little stickers. Thankfully, I guessed the correct row to run down and was able to find my sticker without running past it.

I hung my bike on the rack, threw my helmet under my bike, put on my running shoes, grabbed my race belt, and took off running. As I ran, I fastened my race belt around my waist.

Run

I could hear my coach yelling as I started the run, "Good job, Sue! Drink at *every* water station. The first one is around the corner!" I could hear urgency in his voice, and I knew I needed to listen to what he was saying. The temperature at eighty-four degrees Fahrenheit wasn't too hot, but the humidity was problematic at 94 percent. With the high humidity, less sweat would evaporate from my body. Since sweating is the process through which the body cools itself, it's easy to overheat in humid conditions. If I became dehydrated, my blood would thicken, requiring my heart to beat faster, which would raise my body temperature even more.

Thankfully, Coach Brant had talked to me about this before the race, and we prepared for the heat. During hot Indiana summer days, I did run workouts in the midafternoon, wearing my winter coat and hat. By the time I got to Worlds, my body was used to running in hot and humid conditions, but that didn't eliminate the importance of water during a race. Water was key. Ice was key, too. Coach Brant instructed me to dump ice into my bra if ice was offered at water stations. That would help keep my core temperature down.

As I approached the first water station, I discovered they had ice cubes in cups. I grabbed a cup of ice as I ran and quickly dumped it into my sports bra. I could hear the ice cubes jiggling in my bra as I ran—a ridiculous and wonderful sound. Instead of being in cups, water was provided in sealed baggies. I took two from the volunteers. Coach Brant had shown me how to open the water bags before the race. I grabbed the corner of one packet in my teeth, tore it off, and poured the ice-cold water over my head to further lower my body temperature. Then I bit the corner off a second packet and drank the ice-cold water. All of this was done without stopping or walking. I didn't want to lose any time.

As I started the run, the inside of my right knee began hurting. It had been bothering me a little bit all week, but after a while, the pain went away. Phew! I also felt tired as I started running, but knew I had paced the bike well and should have enough energy to run strong.

The first time I checked the run computer on my wrist, my heart rate was 150 beats per minute. I was supposed to run the first mile with a heartrate of 151, and I was pleased to be so close. I worked to sustain that heart rate—no more, no less. Toward the end of the first mile, I noticed some people were walking in the severe heat. Passing them gave me a boost of confidence. My heat acclimation training was working. I later learned that several people collapsed during the run, due to the scorching temperatures.

My wrist computer indicated that my pace was much slower than it usually is with a 150 heart rate, which I knew was due to the heat. I didn't want to be tempted to run faster, so I stopped monitoring my pace. Instead, I just looked at my heart rate. I knew that everyone would slow in the heat, not just me.

As I approached the one-mile mark, I became more uncomfortable. I was thankful for the pep talk my brother had sent in an email the day before, and I started using his four-beat mantra: *Looking . . . good. . . . More of . . . the same.* Not only did the mantra take my focus to a more positive place, but it felt as though Tom was there with me as I ran.

The second water station was at the one-mile mark. I noticed that all of the ice glasses were empty. At the far end, a man turned from a big cooler with ice in his cupped hands. He was about to place the ice in one of the cups, but I didn't want to wait for that to happen. "Ice!" I yelled. I held the front of my triathlon suit open as I ran by, and leaned forward a little. He knew what I wanted. He lifted his hands and dumped the ice directly into my bra. I saw him laugh. I laughed, too. We would both probably tell that story for years.

After one mile, I struggled a bit more, and my breathing became more labored. I checked my heart rate. It was 153. I was not supposed to go over 155 until the last half mile. I had a mile and a half to run before that point. I needed to be careful. I knew that if my heart rate was over 155 for more than six minutes, my body would slow down, no matter what I told it to do or how hard I pushed. With a mile to go, I checked my heart rate again. Now it was 156—too high, too soon. I was in jeopardy of collapsing before the finish. I slowed my pace, and my heart rate leveled out at 156. I didn't feel desperate, as I had at other times when I pushed too hard, too soon. I figured (hoped) that 156 would be OK. Shortly after that, I saw Coach Brant on the side of the road. He yelled, "Looking good, Sue!" as I ran past.

With three-quarters of a mile to go, my heart rate was at 158, and I was beginning to feel the intense pain that comes from running at a high intensity over time. It's hard to describe that pain. It's not centralized like the pain that comes when you cut yourself or stub your toe. Your body hurts all over—lungs, legs, arms. Your brain's central regulator senses that your body is in trouble, and it begins screaming at you to stop. But I still wasn't feeling desperate, so I decided to ignore the pain and try to sustain my heart rate at 158. I focused on my cadence and willed my legs not to slow down. The course looped back around, and I again saw Coach Brant at the side of the road, "Lookin' good, Sue! Gotta kick it at 2.5 miles!"

When I reached 2.5 miles, I had only a half mile to go. I knew I was supposed to turn up the effort and increase my pace at that point, but I felt horrible. Now I was desperate. I wasn't sure I'd be able to finish. I worried that I had misjudged the situation and should have slowed down when my heart rate went above 155 a quarter mile back. At the pace I was running, my heart rate would be above 155 for more than six minutes. I didn't know if I could make it.

I told myself, *A half mile is just two trips around the high school track back home.* I turned up the effort, although I wasn't sure I had two trips around the track in me. With a quarter mile to go, my heart rate hit 160. That was pretty high. *Just one more trip around the track. Do. Not. Give. In.* I focused on my cadence and commanded my legs not to slow down. I stopped looking at the computer on my wrist. At this point, the data didn't matter. Only my willpower could carry me across the finish line now.

At the turn before the finish chute, I saw Tim Yount, the chief operating officer of USA Triathlon, on the sideline. He was a bigwig, and he was cheering for *me.* "Go, Team USA!" he yelled. That gave me a burst of energy. The finish chute was in sight. My mantra changed: *Just make it that far. Just make it that far. Just make it that far. Keep going!*

Then I was in the finish chute. Just a little farther to the finish arch. *Keep going.* A woman passed me. The number on her calf indicated that she was in a younger age group, but even so, I was determined not to let her beat me to the finish line and somehow found another gear inside me. I gritted my teeth as I chased her down the finish chute. And just before running under the finish arch, I passed her.

Except it wasn't the finish arch. There were two arches. Surprised, I saw another arch in front of me, and it said FINISH across the top of it. The race was not over. The woman passed me again. Once again, I chased her down the finish chute, but this time, I couldn't catch her. She beat me to the finish. But that didn't matter. It was a great race, and I knew I'd given my very best effort.

On the other side of the finish line, I wanted to collapse. Every part of my body screamed for me to put it out of its misery by lying down on the ground, but I knew I had to keep walking to help my body recover. I couldn't stand upright, so I put my hands above my knees to support myself, and I walk-waddled the best that I could.

Medics came rushing up, "Are you OK?" I was breathing so hard that I couldn't answer. A man handed me a bottle of water and put an arm around me for support. "Let's go to the medical tent," he said. He started guiding me toward the tent, but I could finally talk and told him I would be OK. I just needed to walk for a few moments.

The worst part about running a race hard at the finish is that in the finisher photos, I always look like I am about to die. Other people finish with celebratory smiles on their faces and their arms held high in the air in victory as they cross the finish line. But I always look like death. I thought about not running so hard at the end of Worlds; I wanted to grab an American flag and wave it over my head as I finished. But I decided I had come to Worlds to race, so I ran my heart out until the very end. In my Worlds finisher photos, the grimace on my face says it all. I left everything I had on the course.

As I walked away from the finish line, a volunteer placed a finisher's medal around my neck. I was so pleased with all that the medal represented—all the hard work that had gotten me to that point. Then another volunteer handed me a red rose. I walked past food stations, but food didn't sound good at that point.

And then I saw ice baths. Athletes lounged in kid's swimming pools filled with water and ice. I had never taken an ice bath, and the water looked absolutely filthy, but I never thought twice about submerging my beaten, exhausted body into its coolness. I was so hot and miserable that the dirty, icy water looked like a piece of heaven. I laid my medal and rose on the ground next to the little pool and submerged myself to the chin in the delightfully frigid water for a few minutes before going to find Brian and Coach Brant.

The walk to the spot where Brian and Coach Brant stood waiting was special. I thought about the deep hope I'd held at 335 pounds that my life could be different, and I reflected on the tenacity it had taken to stick with my weight loss and training plans. I remembered all the fears I had overcome, all the people who had helped me, and how I had returned to my faith.

When Brian saw me, he snapped a photo as I walked toward him. In the photo, I was too tired to hold my head upright and it leans slightly to my left. My finisher's medal is draped around my neck, and I'm holding my red rose. The smile on my face speaks volumes. It isn't a "woohoo!" smile. It's the smile of someone who has done something incredibly hard and feels deeply satisfied.

In that smile, I also see overwhelming gratitude. For my husband, who supported me every day when I left the house to train, who carried all my gear at races, and who put up with me being too tired to do anything but collapse after hard workouts. For Coach Brant, who saw in me things I didn't see in myself, helped me dream, and then supported those dreams with amazing training plans and talks that built my confidence. For the kindness of my work colleagues who supported my flexed work schedule and eagerly covered for me when I was at races. For friends and perfect strangers who said just the right thing at just the right to time to keep me going. And mostly for God, who had blessed me beyond belief.

Brian, Coach Brant, and I talked about the race for a little bit, and then Brian took photos of Coach Brant and me with an American flag draped around our shoulders. That special moment still fills my eyes with tears. A victorious team of two, we went from 335 pounds to the Age Group Triathlon World Championship.

We had no idea where I had placed in the race. The race officials had not yet posted the results. But I really didn't care about my place. I'd had three process goals for this race. The first was to prepare to the best of my ability. Check. The second was to overcome my fears and make it across the start line. Check. The third was to execute my race plan well and get across the finish line as fast as possible. Check. I was happy with my performance, no matter what.

Finally, the results were posted online. I was eleventh—eleventh in the entire *world*. I flew home with the grandest feeling of satisfaction and wondered what miracles the following year would bring.

TRIATHLON SEASON 5

SIXTH IN THE WORLD

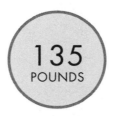

135
POUNDS

Chapter 15

BLUES AND JOYS

After the Age Group Triathlon World Championship in Cozumel, I rode an emotional roller coaster. At times, I was still high as a kite. I couldn't believe I had finished eleventh in the world. Heck, I couldn't even believe I went to Worlds. I cherished all the sweet memories and felt so blessed. But other times, I was terribly sad and lethargic as I started a two-week off season. I still did workouts, but Coach Brant didn't give me a lot of directions. He'd tell me to swim for fun or take a joy ride on my bike. But nothing felt joyous. I felt lost and empty. That made no sense to me, and to be honest, it scared me. What was happening to me? I didn't know what to do.

I did a Google search for "post-race" and "sad" and learned to my surprise that many athletes suffer from sadness after big races. The articles I found even had a name for what I was feeling: post-season blues. Evidently, among people who compete in athletic and other seasonal events, many experience post-season blues. I read articles about post-season blues for triathletes, marathon runners, swimmers, tennis players, and even dog trainers. Post-season blues affect all levels of athletes, from beginners to Olympians. While not everyone gets post-season blues, the condition may be more likely among those who commit seriously to training.

With deep relief, I discovered I wasn't alone and the more I thought about it, the more my feelings started to make sense. For two years, my life had been on full throttle as I focused on doing whatever it took to qualify for Team USA and then race at peak performance at Worlds. Every day except Sundays, I had spent hours training, fueling my body, studying my data, planning, and caring for my equipment. Sleep had become part of my training routine. Exchanging thoughts about the day's workout with Coach Brant had become part of my training routine. For two years, everything I did outside of my job had been focused on preparing for the one point in time when I would race at Worlds.

Then there was the excitement of race week—traveling to another country, meeting athletes from all over the world, wearing my Team USA uniform, and dealing with challenges I couldn't control, like jellyfish, rogue currents, and hot weather. I had lived with intense fear, surging adrenaline, and lots of pressure.

Then it was race day. The air horn blasted. The world stopped. I raced. In the last half mile, I gave every ounce of energy I had left after all the preparation. I ran on fumes and crossed the finish line with the tank on empty.

After the race came more huge emotions. I felt so satisfied. Every day for two years, I had done what I needed to do, and on race day,

I had followed my coach's race plan and held nothing back. I was so happy and excited after the race that I could hardly stand it.

And then suddenly it was over.

• • •

In the aftermath of the race, when the blues first descended, I felt silly. I didn't understand how I could be anything but wildly happy after placing eleventh in the world. It just didn't make sense. But even more than silly, I felt disturbed by what appeared to be a lack of gratitude. It seemed selfish to be in a funk when so many people had believed in me and invested in me. They deserved to see a happy Sue, not a blue Sue. Furthermore, I wondered how I could be in a funk when so many bigger problems existed in the world. I had food to eat, clothes to wear, a roof over my head, and the freedom to pursue my dreams. I had friends and family who loved me. I had my health when others had illness and injury. I had discovered an athletic spirit hiding inside of me and transformed into a healthier version of myself. I was blessed. Worst of all, I knew my funk was not bringing glory to God, who had given me amazing gifts. I wanted to respond with joy and gratitude, but I just couldn't.

As I read more about post-season blues, I was relieved to read that the situation is temporary. In *The Triathlete's Guide to Mental Training*, Jim Taylor, PhD, and Terri Schnider explain that athletes demand a lot from their body over a long period of time, both in training and racing.[1] Once they've met their goal, their body shuts down to recuperate. The authors say that funk is the body's way of shouting, "Give me a rest!" That I understood. I knew I had to be patient and let the blues take their course as I recovered.

It also occurred to me that if I had a new A race on the calendar for the coming season, everything would have purpose again. Even fun runs and joy rides would have purpose, as they helped me recovery mentally and physically in preparation for my next A race. I asked to meet with Coach Brant, and we developed my race schedule for the following season. That helped tremendously. I was back in the groove, as hope for the new season slowly began to replace my post-season sadness.

In November, I raced at the USA Triathlon Draft-Legal World Qualifier in New Orleans. Since I hadn't finished in the top eight at USA Triathlon National Championship during the previous season, I would need to be in the top ten at the World Qualifier to stay on Team USA for another year. The post-Worlds blues were now behind me, and I looked forward to competing at the draft-legal World Qualifier race.

When I arrived at the venue in New Orleans on the morning of the race, I felt prepared and eagerly looked forward to the swim, bike, and run. But as soon as I got out of the car, I learned that the swim portion had been canceled because a fifteen-miles-per-hour wind had created very rough water in Lake Pontchartrain. Instead, the swim would be replaced with a run. So we'd run 3.1 miles, bike for 12.4 miles, and then run again for an additional 1.4 miles. As soon as I heard the news, I was concerned. One of my stronger events was being replaced by one of my weaker events. That was not going to help me place in the top ten. On the contrary, it would help the better runners.

At the start of the run, everyone took off at top speed, but I followed my race plan. I hoped the women in my age group who started out so fast would tire and I'd pass them later. That's exactly what happened. In the third mile, I caught two of them. We were running into the strong wind, and to stay out of the wind, I ran behind them before passing. I couldn't believe what a difference that made. When I came into transition, I knew I'd had a good run because almost all of the other women's bikes were still on the racks.

The bike was a blast. The course was two loops on a relatively flat course. After the first mile, a group of much younger women passed me. They were on their second lap. Instinctively, I pushed to catch them. The group was well organized and impressive to watch. Each woman was taking a forty-five-second pull before dropping to the back. When the first woman came back, she hesitated. I could see her thinking about whether she should come in front of me or behind me. She pulled in front of me. The next woman did the same thing. I thought that was good, because at the back, I was less likely to have to pull at the front. But it was not a good thing.

The woman in front suddenly stood and turned on the gas. All the others did the same and were able to keep with her. But I was taken by surprise. By the time I stood on my pedals, they were out of draft range. I now had a firsthand understanding of what it means to be "spit out the back." I really worked but could not catch them without the benefit of the draft.

A short while later, another group of younger women passed me. One noted my name on my Team USA tri kit and yelled, "Come on, Reynolds," and I was able to have the benefit of the draft with their group.

When I came into transition for the second time, I noticed that all of the bikes for the women my age were gone. I was in first place coming off the bike, with just 1.4 miles of running to go. I hoped the fast runners were far behind and told myself not to get too excited—just follow my race plan.

The second run was different from the first. We ran on the grass up to the levee that would contain the water if Lake Pontchartrain flooded. The grass seemed to have grown in clumps and was very uneven. I was afraid I'd twist an ankle. After about a third of a mile, we were back on pavement. No one passed me. I was still in first place. At around 0.6 miles, a woman passed me. She looked very young, so I didn't think she was in my age group. Shortly after that, we started up a very steep incline to a bridge; she started walking, and I passed her. But on the way back down, she passed me again and stayed in front.

When the results were posted, I found that I had finished in second place. I had led the race until the young-appearing woman passed me during the second run. While she appeared young, she was in my age group. But better than second place, I had qualified for Team USA for a second year and a chance to compete at the Age Group Triathlon World Championship in the Netherlands the following summer. I called Coach Brant to share the news and then stood on the podium as the silver medal was placed around my neck.

• • •

A few days after the race, Coach Brant received devastating news. Karen's chemotherapy hadn't worked. The cancer had grown. Surgery was quickly scheduled. While Karen lay sleeping from the anesthetic, the doctors told Coach Brant that the cancer was worse than they had thought, and they'd had to remove more tissue than anticipated. Coach Brant would have to tell his wife the news when she awoke.

While Coach Brant was my triathlon coach, the way he lived his life taught me much about Christianity. I once asked Coach Brant how he always seemed to know just the right thing to say to people in difficult situations. He responded, "When we do God's work, God gives us the right words to use." Now Coach Brant's choice of words would soften the blow as he told his wife that the cancer was worse than the doctors expected. He later told me it was one of the most difficult things he has ever had to do.

Following surgery, Karen began radiation. When her treatments stopped in February, everyone prayed that the tests results would show no cancer. Those prayers were answered. Karen was, and still is, cancer free. I suspect Coach Brant's and Karen's cancer journey affected many people's faith. It certainly had an impact on mine as I witnessed how their faith gave them peace and strength in such a challenging time.

• • •

I planned to race in the same two A races in the summer of my fifth triathlon season as I had in the previous summer. In August, I would go to Omaha once again for the USA National Championship. Then in September, I'd travel to Rotterdam in the Netherlands to race in my second Age Group Triathlon World Championship.

My annual training plan was similar to previous years' plans. During the fall and winter, I did long, less intense workouts, and then during the spring months, Coach Brant started putting intensity into my workouts. In the summer, I did local races, so Coach Brant could further experiment with pacing and I could get more race experience. And in late July, Coach Brant pushed the intensity sky high during two peak weeks before beginning a one-week taper prior to Nationals.

At Nationals, a new part of my journey began. A few days before the race, a TV reporter from KETV in Omaha called my cell phone to ask if he could interview me. I had been shy about doing interviews, but a few months earlier, a newspaper reporter explained that my story could help others begin their own journey. With that in mind, I agreed to do the interview for KETV as long as it wouldn't distract from my race preparation. We agreed to meet on the dock during swim practice for a brief interview. I told him I would be wearing my bright-green Dream Big Triathlon Coaching triathlon suit.

As I walked down the dock, I saw that a cameraman was already filming me as I approached. Embarrassed, I smiled. The reporter was easy to talk to, like an old friend. As we chatted, the cameraman put the camera right in my face. Then he put the camera on my feet and panned up my entire body. Oh, my. I noticed that people were looking, and I wondered if they thought I was a famous triathlete or maybe an Olympian. I laughed at the thought. No one would mistake *me* for an Olympian.

At the end of the interview, I surprised myself by asking the reporter if he was a Christian. With no sign of surprise or annoyance, he said yes, he was a Christian. I told him about the spiritual side of my journey, and as we talked, the cameraman started filming again. I concluded with, "I know you are doing a public story and can't include the spiritual side." The reporter responded, "Yes, I can."

That evening, Brian and I watched the news in our hotel room. There I was. I felt self-conscious, but at least I didn't sound too goofy. There was no mention of the spiritual side. I imagined that an editor had squelched that part of the story. But later I saw that the reporter had posted about me on his professional Facebook page, where he quoted me talking about God's role in my journey. I had to laugh when I read though all the comments on the report's website. One woman criticized me for being "too skinny." I had never dreamed that anyone would describe me as being too skinny.

Two days later, I competed at Nationals. Although this was my fourth USA Triathlon National Championship, it felt like all the others. I was nervous on the days leading up to the race but strangely calm on race morning. I had trained well all year long and executed my race plan well. When I crossed the finish line, I felt the deep satisfaction that comes with knowing that I had done my best.

One more time, I hoped I would be on the list of the eight people who qualified for Team USA. When the list was posted, I scanned it quickly and saw my name. I was seventh! I was afraid I had misread the list, so I passed it to my husband. "What does this say?" I asked excitedly. He responded, "It says you were seventh!" I would not only be racing for Team USA in Rotterdam later in the summer, but also be racing for Team USA in Australia the following summer. I immediately called Coach Brant to share the news. His excitement filled me with joy. We finally had the outcome that we hoped for after working on our process goals for four years. Finally, a top-eight finish.

The drive from Omaha back home to Indiana was long—nine hours. Along the way, I checked my email and found a message from the Omaha TV reporter. He said a short video about my journey was posted on Facebook. I checked the link and found a thirty-second video about my weight loss and triathlon journey, with footage from the TV interview. A few seconds later, when I went back to the site to send a link to Coach Brant, something seemed wrong: the number of likes was up by five hundred. I refreshed, and the number of likes was up by several hundred more. The video was going viral. I spent the remainder of the drive home refreshing Facebook while laughing with my husband and texting Coach Brant. Five thousand likes! Ten thousand! Two hundred thousand! When the increase in likes finally slowed down, the video had almost three hundred thousand likes, and hundreds of people had shared the video with their Facebook friends. I started wondering if God was giving me opportunities to share the gifts he had given me. The interview with KETV and the video on Facebook were certainly opportunities to share my story. I thought more about using my story to help others and thought a lot about saying just the right words. But then Coach Brant's words came back to me: "When we do God's work, God gives us the right words to use."

• • •

A month after Nationals, Brian and I traveled to Rotterdam so I could race at Worlds. With one world championship behind me, I wasn't as scared about going to Rotterdam as I had been about Cozumel and didn't feel I needed as much hand-holding. So instead of Coach Brant going to Worlds with me, he stayed at home, and we talked daily on the phone as I explored the course and prepared for the race.

I mostly explored the bike course, which was unbelievably technical. The route included thirty-three corners, six hairpin turns, three suspension bridges, four tunnels, cobblestones, and a plywood ramp over a flight of stairs. I felt the technicality of the bike course would work well for me, since I had grown to be rather fearless on the bike. The only part of the bike course that concerned me was the Van Brienenoordbrug Bridge. During the practice ride organized by USA Triathlon, about fifty members of Team USA rode behind the Team USA coach in a cold drizzle. As we approached Van Brienenoordbrug Bridge, I was near the back of the group. Once on the bridge, I noticed there were no curbs. The pavement just stopped in thin air. The only thing separating people from a 230-foot fall was a short guardrail that felt like it was at knee level as I rode on my bike.

Without curbs or solid walls, I couldn't help but see the water 230 feet below when I looked at the road in front of me.

As we approached the top of the bridge, I noticed that one by one, each rider in front of me was being blown off his or her bike at the top of the bridge. Evidently, the structure of the bridge and the direction of the wind were working together to create a crazy-strong wind that blasted around one of the bridge's posts. Needless to say, I jumped off my bike and walked across that point, holding tightly to my bike so it wouldn't blow into the Nieuwe Maas River 230 feet below.

Coach Brant was wonderful each evening as I shared more and more about the course. We worked together as a well-oiled machine as he advised, motivated, and reassured me across the miles. In contrast to my mood in Cozumel, I had no major meltdowns. Emotionally, I had grown over the past year.

On race morning, I left the hotel by myself. My husband had recently had a knee replaced and was unable to accompany me. Instead, he would meet me at the race finish. Unlike the Cozumel procedure, we racked our bikes on race morning instead of the day before. I rode my bike from the hotel to transition with all my gear in cinch bags balanced on my back. I was calm and happy. I was about to do the job I had trained to do.

The race was amazing. Once again, I didn't care where I finished. I just wanted to perfectly execute the plan that Coach Brant had written for me. If I did that, I'd be happy, regardless of where I placed.

The bike portion of the race quickly became one of my favorite triathlon experiences. I loved the challenges of the technical course as we wound our way over and then under the famous Erasmus Bridge and through the streets of Rotterdam. Part of the route took us on narrow bike paths with curbs on both sides. At one point toward the start of the race, as I was passing a woman on a bike path, she pulled too far to the side, and I heard her pedal scrape against the curb. Thankfully, she didn't go down. Instead, she sped up and latched onto my back wheel. We now had a pack of two. Little by little, we passed other women from younger age groups. The stronger ones sped up to join our group, and we were soon riding with women from the USA, Great Britain, and Australia. We were ten-years-old again, riding our bikes through the streets of Rotterdam for the sheer joy of it.

Once again, I took leadership of the group and shouted encouragement to everyone. Our teamwork functioned beautifully. When the race was over, we found each other at the finish line. The bike segment had been just as special for them as it had been for me. We talked excitedly, like ten-year-olds, about all the technical challenges we had faced during the bike segment of the race, and how wonderful it was to work together. Brian found us and took photos of our little group.

As I stood talking, I got a text from Coach Brant. He had been watching a live broadcast of the race on the Internet and sent a photo of me crossing the finish line. His words made my heart sing:

COACH BRANT: Crushed it!! So proud of you.
ME: Thank you, Brant. Those four words mean so much to me!

Brian found the race results online. I was seventh. Seventh in the *world!* I couldn't believe it. As I scrolled through the finishers, I was even more shocked: not only was I seventh, but I was also the first American. I literally shook with excitement as sent Coach Brant a screen shot of the results.

ME: 1ST USA!
COACH BRANT: !!!! 7th in the world!!!!
COACH BRANT: First American! That's incredible!

I called Coach Brant excitedly and shared everything that had happened during the race, babbling good news at a rapid-fire pace. I told him this wasn't *my* success, it was *our* success. We were a team. He wrote the plan that took me from 335 pounds to seventh in the world and first American. I just did what he had told me to do. He was the brain. I was the executor. We had succeeded beyond our wildest dreams.

A few days later, I had another surprise. The race organizers announced that one of the women who had finished in front of me had been disqualified because she "did not finish the course." I was actually sixth in the world. I couldn't believe it.

In the extreme jubilation of the moment, I realized how much I had changed. Five years ago, I couldn't put on my own shoes, and now I put on shoes while racing at twenty miles per hour on a moving bike. Five years ago, I ate a candy bar or an entire package of cookies every time I stopped for gas, and now my favorite foods were yogurt and oatmeal. Five years ago, I was consumed by fears, and now I easily did things that used to scare me, telling pride and fear to go away. Five years ago, I struggled to walk to the neighbor's driveway, and now I was sixth in the world and first American at the Age Group Triathlon World Championship!

• • •

My life has been blessed in so many ways. I am grateful for my family, for Coach Brant, for my friends and colleagues, and the perfect strangers who said just the right thing at just the right moment, and for a loving God who put these gifts in my life and loves me just the way I am. But even now, when I look back, I shake my head in wonder. Even though I witnessed my journey firsthand, it seems unbelievable. But then I realize it is believable. Anything is possible when you have hope for the future, the tenacity to take one little step after another, and the blessings that come with faith. Anything is possible when you have the courage to start a journey—whatever that journey may be.

Note

1. Jim Taylor and Terri Schneider, *The Triathlete's Guide to Mental Training* (Boulder, CO: VeloPress, 2005).